IS BUTTER a CARB?

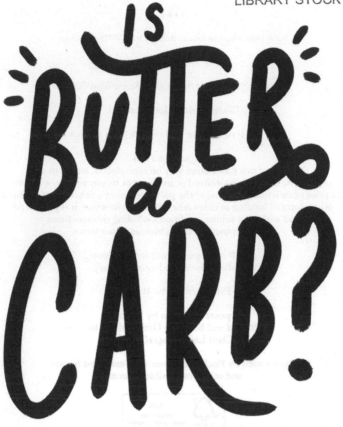

IS BUTTER a CARB?

ROSIE SAUNT and HELEN WEST
The founders of 'The Rooted Project'

piatkus

PIATKUS

First published in Great Britain in 2019 by Piatkus

3 5 7 9 10 8 6 4 2

Copyright © Rosie Saunt and Helen West 2019

Illustrations by John Ratford

The moral right of the authors has been asserted.

A CIP catalogue record for this book
is available from the British Library.

ISBN 978-0-349-41929-9

London EC4Y 0DZ

An Hachette UK Company
www.hachette.co.uk

www.improvementzone.co.uk

The information in this book is not intended to replace or conflict with
the advice given to you by your GP or other health professionals. All
matters regarding your health should be discussed with your GP. The
authors and publisher disclaim any liability directly or indirectly from the
use of the material in this book by any person.

For Enzo and Austin

Contents

Contents

Introduction

We should probably start by telling you that this isn't a regular diet or wellness book. Well, not in the traditional sense anyway. We're not here to talk to you about our 'health journey', cosmic energy, food rules or macro plans, and there's not a recipe in sight. But wait! Before you ditch us for the latest quick-fix diet, you should know that we have something much better than the current food trends in store for you. More than a list of rules, this book will give you a solid grounding in the basics of nutrition and use current scientific understanding to dig through the 'whys' when it comes to the big questions about what to eat.

Finding sensible, practical, evidence-based nutrition advice can be tough going, but as registered dietitians we spend our days trying to offer up precisely that. As co-founders of The Rooted Project – through which we offer up easy to understand nutrition information based on fact, not fads – we spend a lot of our nights organising events to connect the public and nutrition professionals alike, with leading experts on the latest research in nutrition and food science. That's right: our days and nights. That's how much we care.

People have never been more confused about what they should be eating and, as a result, everyone is increasingly looking for information from reliable figures in the nutrition industry to help them pick through the noise. Traditionally, science books can be heavy going; diet books are unrealistic; wellness books lack scientific credibility and tend to embrace brand-building over responsible communication; and evidence-based books are boring. But we believe that this book offers up something new: we're translating the latest research direct to your plate and making evidence-based nutrition accessible and engaging. We're looking to give you a credible resource that will provide you with a solid grounding of knowledge so that you can move forward and make your own decisions about food and how best to fuel yourself. In short, we're talking about empowerment, people, and there's nothing more liberating than that.

Here's the thing. We all know that what we choose to eat can have an impact on our health, but in the seemingly endless sea of conflicting nutrition claims and contradictory advice, it can be near impossible to know how to eat so that we feel and function at our best. Obviously, in all of this we're not short of options. The internet is full of advice. We've got cookbooks and apps and more Insta health gurus than green juices in a yoga barn. But most of us are still walking about wondering things like: would all my problems be solved if I just started food prepping on Sundays? Should I be cutting carbs? Or eating them, but just not the gluten-filled ones? Should I be vegan? Or paleo? Or raw, even? Oh, and while we're at it can someone tell me WTF gluten even is?! And, ultimately, when it comes down to it, is [insert food here] healthy? And should I be eating this?

How is it that the simple act of eating has become such a minefield of paradoxical 'facts'? And when it comes to food, why are most of us left with a profound sense that our diets just aren't 'healthy' enough?

The truth is, there's no one perfect diet for everybody. Eating well is both an art and a science. There's an art to cooking a delicious meal, organising your time, shopping and keeping your food bills within your budget. The science of eating is something different. There is no unassailable set of rules or absolutes. Science is a tool – and a power tool at that. It's a way to cut through all the noise and make sense of the information we're bombarded with daily. It's born of evidence and reason and although it can seem intimidating (and let's be honest, maybe even a little dull), it's something that – with a bit of help – everyone can use and apply to their everyday lives. It can help you shape your diet and give you confidence in your choices, safe in the knowledge that you're basing your decisions on the best current information (and not the latest product or most recent YouTube trend).

You will learn that when it comes to the science of nutrition, things are rarely black and white. They are, instead, several wonderfully interesting shades of grey. So let us talk you through this fascinating science and teach you how you can harness its power to find a sustainable diet that's right for you.

1

What's the Harm?

The way we eat has changed dramatically over the last two generations. On the one hand, we are lucky enough to live at a time when food in the UK is plentiful, even if it's not, unfortunately, always affordable for everyone. On the other, for those of us privileged enough to be able to take advantage, the abundance of choice, coupled with the wealth of conflicting information about food, can be overwhelming. To add to this perfect storm, we now live in the age of the social media celebrity. This is an era where beautiful twenty-somethings can rise to superstar status, some with little more than a great body, shiny hair and a flashy smile. Our collective cultural desire to be thin and beautiful has gradually seen us turn to an industry preoccupied with youth and aesthetics, not only to tell us where to go, what to do and how to dress, but also how to eat. 'Eat like me, look like me' has become the unspoken mantra of the wellness industry. And while on the surface all the green juices, flexed abs and artfully arranged smoothie bowls look like they should be contributing to the greater good and improving our overall health, when you dig a bit deeper the waters start to muddy a little.

That is how we find ourselves where we are now – knee

deep in the backlash against diets and 'clean eating'. People are angry. And rightly so. In the current nutrition climate, diets are seen as 'so last season', but labels still rule. Lifestyles such as veganism, carnivore, paleo and keto have become the new religions, amassing tribes of followers and creating communities based around the food that people choose (or, more accurately, choose not) to eat. And while clean eating may be on its way out, there's always something to take its place. Heard of 'Real Food', anyone? There are also whole websites dedicated to presenting 'alternatives' and scaremongering about the food we eat, usually to support an individual narrative or collective agenda. Even communities whose dietary choices are driven by a desire to eat in a sustainable and ethical way are occasionally guilty of engaging in dubious propaganda about their diets' health benefits. A common vegan argument levelled against cow's milk, for example, is that we (humans) are the only species to consume another species' milk. This is usually accompanied by a list of 'facts' designed to shock, including a recent favourite that cow's milk contains trillions of 'pus cells'. But neither story tells the whole truth. The bigger picture is that while it's true that humans are the only species to drink another species' milk, we are also the only species to do a lot of things – like cook, go to restaurants or buy books from a bookshop. We're socially and developmentally advanced and therefore have opportunities when it comes to sourcing our food that other species do not. That's not to say our broader food industry is unimpeachable by any means, but the isolated fact of humans participating in a nutrition activity not seen in other animals does not in itself tell us anything at all, especially about health. As for 'pus cells', this is just a non-scientific way of describing white blood cells. It's a term that elicits groans of 'ewwww' (which, of course, is precisely why it has been chosen) but it's a very normal part of any mammal's milk. Using the term in this way, you could also say that human milk contains trillions of pus cells, but we're guessing you'd still give it to your baby.

The crux of the issue is this: eating is a field in which everybody can claim expertise – we do it every day. But as the number of social media accounts dedicated to diet and health increase and continue to amass thousands of followers, vast swathes of the public are getting their dietary advice from these sorts of anecdotes and conspiracies over and above scientific evidence.

It all sounds a bit bleak when you put it down on paper like this, but it's a stark reality. Obviously, not everybody talking about nutrition on the internet is doing a bad job – and many of the people out there spreading their messages about food have good intentions, even if they aren't quite hitting the mark with their content. That said, anecdotes can be incredibly powerful, especially when they're coming from somebody that you feel you know, trust and admire. As a result, at The Rooted Project we believe that people with significant influence and social media followings have an ethical responsibility to their audience to get it right, especially when they are doling out nutritional advice, and that, when it comes to food, using a system of logic and reason (oh, hi science!) rather than opinion, is crucial.

Unfortunately, as all qualified nutrition professionals have come to know, using scientific research to point out the potential harm in some of the messages generated by these communities – from 'eat clean' to 'grains are toxic' – can be seen as nit-picking. As a nation, we eat too much sugar and not nearly enough vegetables or fibre, so is it necessary to pick people up on what might seem to be minor indiscretions? If health bloggers and Insta celebs spout a bit of nutrition nonsense but are inspiring people to eat more vegetables and pay attention to their diet, surely that's a good thing? Maybe even the most important thing, if we want to improve the nation's health. And does it really matter if people have the right qualifications and training?

This is something we've heard a lot since people have started to criticise the internet for its endless stream of nutri-bollocks.

So let's take a step back and explore this.

The idea that food can help us on our way to good health isn't unfounded. We know that, in general, people who consume diets rich in fruits and vegetables, and who choose whole foods, including good-quality carbohydrates, fats and proteins, are less at risk of disease than those who don't.[1] [2] But the idea that nutrition in a vacuum is responsible for our health status, or that there's one perfect diet out there for all of us and that the inclusion (or exclusion) of specific foods in our diets will, without fail, protect us from ill health, is, unfortunately, nonsense. This message is part of the subtext of the diet and wellness industry (which are really one and the same), and it's harmful. In its essence, the pursuit of maintaining good health and being well is a wonderful idea, but when you dress it up in expensive clothes and stick a label on it, it becomes little more than a fancy (often elitist) diet. By that, we mean that this approach to health makes it seem as if healthy food is an exclusive and elusive commodity, available only to the elite, 'enlightened' few.

Take Elle Macpherson's Super Elixir powder: this greens powder, according to Elle's nutritionist, improves your 'inner fitness, supports nutrition at a cellular level and optimises the functioning of all 11 systems of the human body'. It contains 46 ingredients, costs an eye-watering £96 for a month's supply and implies that if you aren't adhering to the lifestyle they recommend you can expect a body which isn't functioning at its best.

Likewise, Amanda Chantal Bacon (of LA-based Moon Juice fame) sells her cleverly branded and beautifully packaged herbal supplements (from 'Brain Dust' to 'Action Powder') as neatly packed solutions to modern-day problems. These powders also come with an impossibly obscure ingredients list and a hefty price tag – a standard in this industry dominated by the wealthy-but-worried middle class – and when you use privilege to exploit a collective cultural neurosis in this way, a healthy life can end up seeming profoundly out of reach for many of us. Further to this idea – that in order to safeguard your health you need to have a perfect diet, detox regularly and take an unfathomable amount of expensive supplements – there is a general unspoken suggestion in the wellness industry that any ill health is entirely your own doing. Got cancer? Probably all that [insert food stuff here] you were eating. Got a sore tummy? It's probably all those toxic carbs (and not because it's that time of the month).

The harm caused by these confusing nutrition messages, of course, occurs on a sliding scale.

At the lower end of this spectrum, the harm is principally that people waste money on rubbish products, diets or foods that they don't really need and which don't live up to the hype. Have you ever been out and spent a butt-load of money on a magic nutrition 'pill' or food product which claimed it would help you to lose weight/have more energy/detoxify your body, only to find that once the initial buzz of using said product has worn off, the effects it promised haven't actually materialised? This sort of thing isn't usually a danger to your health, but it does trick you into feeling like you need to invest in special foods or products to make your diet healthier, and it's certainly harmful to your wallet.

For example, supplement spending is on the rise in the UK, with global market research estimating Britons spend £400 million on vitamins and supplements each year. The daily use of vitamins and minerals has increased from 41 per cent in 2015 to 46 per cent in 2016,[3][4] meaning that almost half the UK take vitamins and minerals despite little evidence that (unless you are deficient) they carry any health benefits. It can also be damaging to the mental health of people who buy into the negative messages about the latest demonised food, especially if they can't afford the special alternatives popularised by bloggers and influencers. How would you feel as a parent who believes that because you're not able to feed your family unaffordable organic produce, you're exposing them to highly toxic 'synthetic' pesticides? For a person trying to do the best for their children, these seemingly harmless messages can be the cause of a lot of angst and stress.

Moving onwards up the scale, some of the physical health effects of misinformation about nutrition start to emerge. Scaremongering about food groups from carbohydrates to specific nutrients, such as gluten, can cause such confusion that people unnecessarily cut them from their diet, out of fear that they are toxic and cause disease. Not only does this mean that people are shunning perfectly healthy foods, but it can also result in damaging changes to both diet and body. It's known, for example, that unnecessarily following a gluten-free diet can reduce the amount of fibre and micronutrients such as calcium and vitamin B12 that you consume.[5] Likewise, following a low-FODMAP (Fermentable Oligosaccharides, Disaccharides, Monosaccharides and Polyols – otherwise known as carbohydrates) diet (which is prescribed therapeutically to help identify dietary triggers of irritable bowel syndrome) over a long period has been shown to reduce numbers and types of good bacteria in your gut – which may affect your long-term health.[6] The powerful belief that some foods are 'good' and others are 'bad' can contribute to a complicated and turbulent relationship with food and potentially even orthorexia, the term used to describe an anxious obsession with purity in pursuit of a healthy diet.[7] Currently we categorise having a poor relationship with food as a 'medium risk', but the resulting behaviours can have a serious impact on both your mental and physical health. This is something we'll be discussing in more detail later, as we explore diet culture and the concept of intuitive eating.

On the extreme end of the scale you have people putting their lives at risk by rejecting proven medical therapies in favour of diet as a 'cure-all'. 'Food as medicine', as people like to say, sounds logical, but when taken in a literal sense this is a real concern and one that was brought into sharp focus a few years ago when the health blogger and cancer patient Jessica Ainscough, publicly known as 'The Wellness Warrior', passed away. Aged just 22, Jessica was tragically diagnosed with a rare form of soft tissue cancer, called epithelioid sarcoma, in her left arm. Facing the awful reality of her condition and disillusioned with the extreme treatments recommended to manage her cancer, Jessica (perhaps understandably) turned to alternative therapies and used her blogging platform, The Wellness Warrior, to document her journey and advise others. In particular, she promoted the use of Gerson therapy (an intensive dietary treatment regime that includes a strict organic and vegetarian diet, supplements and coffee enemas, which has no scientific evidence to support it) over the advised route of surgical amputation and chemotherapy. Jessica's tale is well-documented and we won't go into it in detail here, but in essence, both Jessica and her mum (who chose a similar treatment route to her daughter to treat her potentially curable breast cancer) were victims of nutritional pseudoscience. They both sadly died of their diseases in the timeframe anticipated for their untreated cancers.

The heartbreaking likelihood is that Jessica's blog, social-media platforms and books persuaded other people with treatable cancer to follow an oncology plan based solely on 'natural' therapies. Similarly, Belle Gibson, another health blogger who claimed to have cured her cancer by diet alone, sold millions of books and had a number one best-selling app with her brand, The Whole Pantry. It later transpired that she had lied and had never had cancer at all.

Obviously, when it comes to healthcare, people should always have autonomy over their own treatment and diet is an important (sometimes vital) part of a treatment plan, but it certainly doesn't have to be one or the other. We'll never know how many people chose Belle and Jessica's treatment routes over medical therapies that might have saved their lives. Thankfully, completely rejecting proven medical therapies in favour of a purely alternative route is rare, but it does happen. The potential effects of this were seen quite clearly in a study conducted by Yale School of Medicine.[8] Scientists observed a group of people undergoing cancer treatment; following either conventional therapy or a solely alternative route (this meant using alternative treatments such as acupuncture or tai chi, which didn't run alongside any conventional therapy). Interestingly, the people choosing alternative treatments were more likely to be younger women, with higher levels of income and education. But even after controlling for other factors that could skew the results, such as age and background, at five years, researchers found that the risk of death was 23 per cent higher in the people who chose alternative therapies compared with those who took a conventional route. In fact, of the women who had breast cancer, those choosing alternative treatments had more than a fivefold increased risk of death at five years. This type of study can't 'prove' that the people who chose alternative therapies would have lived longer if they had taken a conventional route, but the results certainly suggest that their chances of surviving longer would have been greater, even if they had they followed conventional therapies alongside their complementary ones.

The reasons why people choose to believe unqualified celebrities over qualified experts is a complex mix of economic, social, psychological and neurological theory, but two of the more interesting principles that go some way to explaining this phenomenon are 'meaning transfer' and the 'halo effect'. Quite simply, meaning transfer is a marketing theory that predicts that we will view a product in the same light as the person selling it. So, for example, if a celebrity (for ease, let's consider Jessica Ainscough again) is perceived as vibrant, attractive, healthy and successful, people may automatically transfer their belief about that person to a product (or in Jessica's case, a lifestyle), making it more desirable. This is a tactic commonly used by marketers to make their products seem socially aspirational and is one of the many reasons why they covet social media influencers for product endorsements.

The halo effect is a similar phenomenon, but it is even more relevant when it comes to thinking about why people take nutrition advice from celebrities rather than experts. This comes into play when the admiration we feel for a person who we rate positively in one area is extended to include other characteristics. If you see your favourite celebrity as attractive, trustworthy and kind, you are often also likely to believe them to have an array of other positive characteristics, for example, to be clever and knowledgeable, even if they're discussing a field in which they have no expertise.[9] When deployed responsibly, this can be an incredibly powerful and effective public health conduit to offer up good advice. Jamie Oliver's hugely successful Ministry of Food campaign notably managed to capture the attention of government officials and his efforts led to the improvement of school food standards across the UK. But if the advice is unsubstantiated or spurious, things have the potential to become dangerous very quickly.

And that's where we come in! Our mission is to ensure that as many people as possible are equipped with the information they need to get a handle on their own health. All considered, the bottom line is this: if you're making your choice based on anecdotes, misleading propaganda and misinformation rather than facts and figures, it suddenly doesn't seem like much of a choice at all, does it?

So, there is a reason why we're coming out strongly against, unaccountable, unsupported dietary information – because all the way up and down that sliding scale there *is* inherent harm in nutri-bollocks. And no matter how appealing the latest superfood or magical supplement seems, you can't ever be empowered by misinformation.

But it's not all bad news. There is an alternative and something we can all do to make things better: we need to start demanding facts, transparency and rigorous professionalism from the people who dispense our dietary advice. We can all do this simply by asking for evidence. So if you're ready to learn about food without the pretence, the judgement or the fads, you're in the right place. We're here to talk you through what we, as a scientific community, do know about diet and health (and what we don't). We're going to teach you how to pick through the non-sense, how to ask for evidence and ultimately give you all the information you need to help you find a way of eating that's right for you – based on fact, not fiction.

2

Calories

Calories. You've almost certainly heard of them. They're everywhere we turn – listed on food packets, highlighted on restaurant menus and even tracked on your smartphone. Often framed as the 'bad guys', most of public health policy is shaped around encouraging us to keep them in check by counting them, minimising them and burning lots of them. Subconsciously, we can even fear them. But what exactly are clories and how many do we need?

What are calories and how are they measured?

We need energy to sustain life; to keep warm, to think, to grow and to be active. And calories (or, more accurately, kilocalories) are the units we use to describe our body's energy budget. We extract calories from food during digestion and use them to go about our daily functions – from doing a downward dog to typing on our laptop or running for the bus. We also use calories (albeit slightly fewer of them) when we are sitting still or sleeping. They keep our hearts beating, our lungs breathing and our brains orchestrating all the complex functions that our bodies organs undertake to keep us alive. So calories are kind of important.

Nutrition scientists have developed a way to measure the calories in food by burning it in a 'bomb calorimeter'. This contraption measures change in water temperature, making it pretty straightforward to calculate the number of calories in a food: if the water temperature goes up by 1 degree per gram, the food sample has 1 calorie; 5 degrees per gram would mean 5 calories, and so on.

One calorie is the amount of energy it would take to raise the temperature of 1 gram of water by 1 degree Celsius.

However, (although it's probably stating the obvious) our bodies are not bomb calorimeters! We (thankfully) don't ignite food inside our stomachs to release fuel, we use chemicals like digestive enzymes and the mechanical motions of chewing and digestion to manipulate food and extract what we can. But it's not a perfect system. As food moves along our digestive tract, our body is unable to squeeze out every available calorie and some of them are then lost into our faeces or our urine. Nutrition scientists have tried to correct for this difference by coming up with some adjusted figures called Atwater factors and it's these values that are used to calculate the calories you see on the food labels of packaged foods in your local supermarket. The most calorie dense nutrients are fats, at 9 calories per gram. Carbs and protein have slightly less at 4 calories per gram and alcohol sits in the middle, with 7 calories per gram.

How many calories do you need?

You've probably heard the government's party line on calories, which is that a man should eat approximately 2500 calories and a woman 2000 calories per day. These estimates are based on average weight, muscle mass and physical activity levels and form the basis of the UK guidelines, so they seem legitimate. But it's not that straightforward. The complexity of our bodies and lifestyles means that although public health guidelines can have a crude stab at guessing what an average person needs, at a personal level the number can vary quite dramatically. The exact number of calories that you require daily (often referred to as your metabolic rate), actually depends on lots of different factors, including your weight, height, sex, age, genetics and body composition. It's also a fluid thing; it can fluctuate depending on how active you are during a particular time, or if other things are going on within your body, such as illness or pregnancy.

Talking point: brain energy

Our brain is a hungry organ and providing it with enough fuel is essential to keep us alive! Considering it makes up a teeny 2 per cent of our total body weight, it consumes a relatively large amount of calories (or energy).[1] With no fuel storage facility, it needs to be supplied with its preferred fuel source (a sugar called glucose) continuously. In fact, it's said the brain uses around 20 per cent of the energy we consume, which research estimates amounts to about 120g glucose per day, the equivalent of about 540 calories or 23 Medjool dates.[2]

Your metabolism

Your metabolism (or metabolic rate) is the umbrella term for all the chemical reactions that occur in your body to keep it functioning. All these processes require energy – or calories.

Although the exact number of calories you need to process these reactions can be influenced by some of the things mentioned earlier, your requirements can be divided up into a few components; your resting energy expenditure (this is the number of calories you require to facilitate all the chemical reactions that take place when your body is at rest); the number of calories used during digestion (known as the thermic effect of food); and the amount of energy needed to fuel your activity through the day.[3]

Can you boost your metabolism?

Our cultural obsession with aesthetics means that there are all manner of pills, foods and products out there that claim to boost your metabolism and make your body burn more calories. But is it really possible to increase your metabolic rate with food or supplements?

Some experimental studies have found that things like drinking coffee and green tea can increase metabolic rate, but only by really tiny amounts that in 'real life' aren't likely to have any meaningful or lasting effects on the amount of calories your body uses.

From a supplement perspective, there are lots out there that claim to burn fat. They usually contain a mixture of ingredients, the main ones touted for their metabolism-boosting effects

▶

being caffeine, green tea extract and raspberry ketones. Although caffeine can temporarily raise your metabolic rate, it's thought that this effect can wear off over the long term as tolerance increases.[4] This isn't the case for green tea extract, which has been proven not to have any effect on your metabolic rate,[5][6] or raspberry ketones, which seem to have a minor effect when taken in *really* high doses in rats but haven't been shown to have much promise of effects in people.

In the fitness industry fat burners that claim to boost your metabolism are often advertised as something that can help you achieve your 'goals'. There has been a rise in deaths associated with the banned fat burner dinitrophenol (DNP): supplements containing DNP have dangerous effects on metabolic rate. They can raise body temperature above the normal range and cause side-effects including an irregular heartbeat, coma and death. These supplements, avowing to be a 'wonder slimming aid', are illegally distributed on the internet and tens of vulnerable people to date have fallen prey to their falsified claims and died as a result of use.[7] Steer clear!

Is a calorie a calorie?

Advocates of specific dietary approaches, most often ones that eliminate certain foods or nutrients, love asking this question: is a calorie a calorie, regardless of provenance or composition? It's a particularly popular line of enquiry when pitting one diet against another, in the hope of 'proving' that the inclusion/exclusion of calories from specific macronutrients will influence health. But is this true?

When people talk calories, they are usually talking about

energy balance and they are usually oversimplifying: e.g. 'calories in, calories out'. It's true that if we look at calories in isolation, as a form of energy, a calorie is a calorie. Lots of studies examining the effect of calories on weight agree on this, from complex and expensive metabolic ward studies conducted by scientists, to self-experiments where people have demonstrated short-term weight loss via calorie-restricted diets of biscuits and cake or fast food (to name just a few). In simplistic terms, then, calories obey the first law of thermodynamics (energy can be neither created or destroyed, only transformed from one form to another), so calories are simply a transfer of energy from the food we eat, into our bodies.[8] So, is that it? Case closed? Not quite. Thinking of calories in this way suggests that the source of your calories doesn't matter (the subtext being that the only thing that matters is your weight). For health, this is both untrue and unhelpful. It's obvious, really: 100 calories' worth of avocado offers much more variety in terms of nutrients than 100 calories' worth of Smarties. And it's just as obvious that sometimes the nutrient content of an avocado really isn't going to hit the spot and only Smarties will do! But by shifting the focus onto *only* calories, we can lose this nuance in the discussion about food and health. When it comes down to it (as we'll be exploring a lot throughout this book) context matters.

A calorie is a calorie. But it's not *just* about calories. For scientists, a calorie is a useful energy measure but, as we've established, working out how many of them each of us requires is highly individualistic. The calorie content of any given food also tells us nothing about what nutrients it contains, or whether our food choices will fill us up or satisfy us. So, in isolation, without the context of the what, why and how the calories are being consumed in the real world, the meaning of the calorie count of foods tells us a very limited amount.

Does caffeine give me energy?

Caffeine is mostly consumed via coffee (as it's derived from the coffee bean), but it's also found in tea, energy drinks, chocolate and cola. Caffeine is actually classed as a 'nootropic', a term for a supplement that is ingested specifically for its effects on the brain. It's thought that caffeine blocks receptors in the brain that promote sleepiness[9] and other receptors in the brain which, when blocked, produce dopamine (a chemical messenger of the nervous system) that has stimulating and mood-enhancing effects.[10] There is also an ongoing debate over whether the effects of caffeine are actually due to dependency: i.e. the caffeine 'boost' that people feel is simply the result of feeling 'back to normal' after a period of caffeine withdrawal, such as an overnight sleep, as opposed to the effects being an improvement from the norm (e.g. 'My morning coffee makes me feel even better than normal'). Luckily for coffee addicts, some recent human trials testing mood and cognition in caffeine and non-caffeine drinkers have suggested this is not the case.[11] So caffeine doesn't give you energy, not in the literal sense anyway (it doesn't contain any calories). But it can make you feel more awake and maybe even improve your mood!

Metabolic adaptation and the 500-calorie deficit myth

Amongst many other misconceptions, the oversimplification of weight loss has led to the common assumption that since there are approximately 3,500 calories in 450g (1lb) of fat, if you increase or decrease your calorie intake by 500 calories per day, you will gain or lose 450g (1Ib) of body fat per week. In other words, if we simply cut calorie intake, we can add up these energy deficits over time, leading to progressive body weight loss, which happens in a linear fashion, pound after pound, day after day. But as anyone who has been on a diet to lose weight knows, in reality this does not happen, especially over the longer term.

What's the reason for this? Despite the common belief that weight loss is simply a matter of cutting calories through will-power and discipline, the reality is much more complex. In times gone by, when food was less readily available and people had to endure periods without eating, rapid weight loss would have been a disadvantage. Naturally, our bodies have evolved mechanisms to defend our weight and protect us from starvation. Collectively the changes to your metabolism during a period of calorie restriction (aka dieting) are known as 'metabolic adaptation' or, in more nerdy circles, 'adaptive thermogenesis'.[12] The first way our body adapts to calorie restriction is by conserving energy in essential functions. When calories are scarce, your body lowers its resting metabolic rate so that it burns fewer calories day to day: essentially, we start to use up less energy when we're sitting on the sofa than we usually would. At the same time, it increases our drive to eat by changing the balance of hormones that are linked to appetite; it's well known that people who are losing weight on a diet experience an increase in ghrelin (also known as the hunger hormone) as well as a decrease in leptin, a hormone linked to body fat that suppresses your appetite. These changes can lead to real, almost unconscious increases in food intake, driven by your biology. One group of scientists wanted to try to quantify this and measure how much more people were likely to eat while in a calorie deficit. To do this they had to design a study in which people weren't consciously following a diet in order to make the results mimic the unconscious, biological adaptations as closely as possible (and reduce the chance that changes in people's food intake were due to the psychological effects of dieting and deprivation). The resulting study was a double-blind, randomised, placebo-controlled trial in which participants either took a placebo or a drug. The people who took the drug unknowingly lost around 360 calories from glucose in their urine per day, putting them into a calorie deficit. Unsurprisingly, they found their bodies adapted to the calorie deficit and their calorie intake increased, by around 100 calories per day for every kilogram of weight they lost.[13]

But how does this play out in real life? The effects of metabolic adaptation are thought to persist for a while after weight loss, explaining why many people who lose weight on a diet then regain most of their weight over the longer term (conservative estimates put this phenomenon at around 80 per cent of dieters[14]). The most striking example we have of this is in the Biggest Loser study. Although an extreme example of metabolic adaptation, it clearly shows the biological capability of the human body to adapt to dieting. *The Biggest Loser*, an American reality TV show, sees people who are classified by the BMI scale as 'morbidly obese' participate in a televised intensive diet and exercise programme and compete to see who loses the most weight. The weight losses are usually large and dramatic. Contestants undertake around 90 minutes of exercise per day, six days a week and eat low-calorie diets of around 1200 calories per day, resulting in losses of up to 60 per cent of their body weight over seven months. If it sounds hellish, we think many past contestants would agree with you. However, what the reality show does demonstrate is the potential long-term after-effects of dieting on the metabolism. A group of scientists interested in the idea of metabolic adaptation spotted this show as an opportunity to conduct some research, and so they followed a group of participants from the Biggest Loser for six years. As expected, immediately after the competition and at the height of their weight loss, the contestant's metabolism was suppressed. Also as expected, over the next six years, participants regained at least some of the weight they had lost. But what surprised the scientists the most was that their metabolisms never seemed to fully recover. When they started the competition, contestants had 'normal' metabolic rates (or burned the number of calories you would expect for somebody of their age and weight). Six years after the competition, participants were burning on average around 500 calories less than they would be expected to for their weight. Weight is influenced by a complex number of factors including your genetics, social status and the environment you live in (to name a few), but as you can imagine, these types of changes make both linear weight loss (as championed by the '500 calories a day' myth) and keeping weight off in the long term, difficult.

Does when you eat your calories matter?

Don't eat after 8pm because all the food you eat will turn to fat. Ever heard this? It's a common saying (which isn't true), but like many of these myths there is a thread of science running through it that has been bent and stretched out of shape to form this classic piece of nonsense.

Let's break this down.

Physiologically, your body stores energy it hasn't used as fat. The how and why this comes to be is complex, but this isn't a process that kicks in at a certain time of day or night.

However, there is a very new and exciting area of research that could explain where this myth came from (we're feeling more generous than 'somebody just made it up', which to be

▶

honest is also a strong possibility) – and that's the study of Chrononutrition.[15]

All our body's cells work to a natural biological rhythm – your body clock is a real thing! – and chrononutrition is the study of how food affects these rhythms (and how this can impact on our health). In its simplest form, your body has two 'clocks': your central clock, which is mainly regulated by light and dark (night and day); and your peripheral clock, which can be influenced by food and nutrients. These clocks run a distinct 24-hour cycle and regulate basically everything, from your organ function to your metabolism. They work to a consistent rhythm, anticipating daily events (like eating and sleeping) and keeping your body working efficiently.

However, because your body's circadian rhythms can be affected by what you eat, erratic eating patterns can mess them up, knocking your body clock out of alignment and disrupting the 'flow' of your metabolic rhythm. This is something you experience in a very real way when you travel across time zones and you feel jet-lagged – that's your body clock all out of whack.

In addition to this, emerging research suggests that we have a more efficient metabolism in the early part of the day (which, roughly speaking, is from when you wake up until around 3pm).[16][17]

And this is where this myth *kind of* fits. Because our bodies are better primed to deal with food in the earlier part of the day, it's been suggested that the old saying 'breakfast like a king, lunch like a prince and dinner like a pauper' might hold some merit. (Especially given this is kind of the opposite of usual eating patterns in the UK, where dinner tends to be the

▶

main meal of the day.) Research into shift workers backs up this line of thought, with studies examining the effects of regular overnight working (and eating out of alignment with your central day/night clock) finding real metabolic consequences that are thought to have a direct impact on health and increase the risk of diseases like diabetes.[18]

But wait! Before you trot off and start determinedly planning dinner parties that finish by 7.59pm, there is no conclusive evidence that points to a **best** time to eat and we still have a lot more to learn about this area before we can make any firm recommendations. What really seems to matter for now is *routine.* So, no, any calories eaten after 8pm won't just be stored as fat, but avoiding skipping meals and eating at regular times through the day could help keep your body's internal clocks happily running on time.

To track or not to track?

One of the things that has dramatically changed over the last decade is the ease with which it is now possible to monitor your calorie intake. Gone are the days where only the most dedicated dieter, armed with a pocket guide to calories and a calculator, was able to tot up their intake. Now smartphone use is a part of everyday life, with an estimated 70 per cent of us in the UK (and rising) owning a device.[19] This means that alongside the raft of wellness apps that allow you to collect everyday data about yourself, apps containing the nutrient and calorie content of thousands of foods are now available at our fingertips, many of them for free. But is this a good thing? Should we be taking advantage of these apps and religiously tracking our calories?

Calorie counting is a controversial topic in the world of nutrition, which plays into the (mostly useless) arguments about which diet is 'best'. Anecdotally, some rave about calorie-counting apps, claiming them to be the holy grail of dieting success. Others state plainly that calorie counting is useless (but recommend tracking macronutrients, i.e. the amount of carbs, proteins and fats, instead, or following a specific dietary pattern like low-carb, high-fat). Finally, the last camp believes using them is a surefire way to promote disordered relationships with food.

Although the number of studies examining these apps has increased significantly over the last few years, it remains an unregulated industry and the amount of information we have on their effects is still pretty limited (with many of the study methods criticised for being of poor quality, or loaded with bias).[20] [21] [22] However, these apps have been under fire for their high dropout rates, too – it's estimated that around 90 per cent of people who download health apps use them once or twice and never log in again. Many others drop off after the first month of usage. Psychologists have also criticised the lack of robust behaviour-change techniques (meaning they aren't set up for promoting long-term changes to habits and behaviours) – all adding up to a big question mark over their usefulness and, more importantly, safety.[23] [24] [25] Safety is indeed one of the main concerns for calorie-counting apps, which have been linked with the onset of eating disorders[26]. Additionally, in one study of more than 100 individuals with a diagnosed eating disorder, 75 per cent reported using calorie trackers, and 73 per cent of them felt that this directly contributed to their eating disorder behaviours.[27]

If you're a person who uses or is thinking about using a tracking app, it is definitely worth weighing up the potential risks against the perceived benefits. On the one hand, tracking apps may seem to be helpful as a source of information and a stepping stone to learn more about your eating habits. They are simple to follow and easy to use. But it's important to be aware that many people find tracking unsustainable and that the lack of flexibility in the calorie prescriptions in these apps may send you into a cycle of unsuccessful dieting. Calorie counting and fitness tracking has also been linked with dietary restraint – which is a risk factor for developing disordered eating.[28] [29]

If you already use a calorie tracker, we'd suggest thinking critically about your relationship with it (and your other health-related apps on your phone). Are these things that you might look at occasionally and can be flexible with? Or are they something that you are dependent on and you find yourself checking several times a day, with the results impacting on both your mood and your social life? On balance, for some, calorie counting can be a tool to identify behaviours that might not be serving them well and encourage them to make healthy changes, but for many this can be harmful, directing the focus away from our body and internal cues and towards a reliance on external data, which, in susceptible people, can result in disordered eating patterns.[30] [31] At their heart, apps like this are deeply binary in their approach to eating. They can't predict natural fluctuations in appetite, which can occur for a vast array of reasons, from a particularly active day to your menstrual cycle.[32] Crucially, it is possible to focus on healthy behaviours and eating habits *without* tracking calories – something we will touch on later in this book when we discuss the process of intuitive eating.

3

Fats

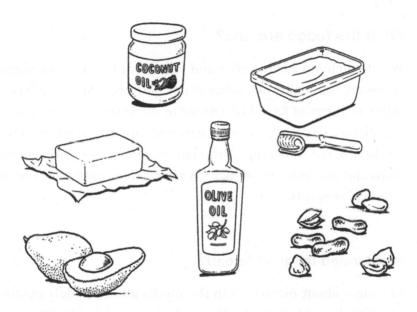

We don't know if you've heard, but fat is *back*, people, and in a big way. Previously considered public health enemy number one due to the suggested link between saturated fat and heart disease, its reprieve has been one of the biggest shake-ups to nutrition science this decade. So much so that low-carb, high-fat diets have now moved firmly out of the realm of 'fad diets' and are considered a mainstream dietary choice. In fact, people are now so convinced of the benefit of fats that they are happily advising you to eat coconut oil by the spoonful and add butter to your coffee (wait, what?). However, despite the advances in our knowledge, the simplification and misrepresentation of the messages about fat to suit different agendas have left us, again, on baffling ground. Is fat healthy or dangerous? Is it high in calories? What sort of fat should we be eating for good health? Should we be fearful of fat or using it liberally to manage our health and our weight? Let's roll right back to the beginning and take a look.

What the fudge are fats?

We often clump fats together and talk about them as one singular entity, but really, like other major nutrients, there are lots of different types of fats. The fats we're interested in in this book are 'dietary fats' (aka, ones we eat) and how they can influence our health and wellbeing. Although avocados, croissants, bacon, chips and almonds are all high-fat foods, their individual contribution is very different.

Is saturated fat good or bad?

Messages about dietary fat in the media are extremely confusing. This is partly because dietary fats are not simple structures to research, and partly because they come in a lot of different forms in lots of different foods. This complexity has meant that since they became implicated in heart disease risk, researchers have spent decades and decades trying to narrow down their role in supporting or harming health. Translating this research into meaningful, practical information for the public can be challenging, as messages risk being too simplistic (and missing the point) or too complex (and being overwhelming). The most important thing to note, though, was that for almost 40 years the public was recommended to follow a diet that was low in fat, due to the links found between saturated fat and heart disease. Although this was straightforward advice, we now know it had unintended consequences, not because following a diet low in fat is 'bad', or because we should all be eating more saturated fat, but because the balance of your whole diet is what is important for health and, most importantly, when you reduce the amount of one nutrient in your diet, what you replace it with matters.

If you're confused about this, don't worry, you're not alone. In the public domain, this is currently one of the most hotly debated topics in nutrition. It's a complicated matter, fraught with nuance and plagued by media narratives that ignore the complexities of the topic and don't quite give the full picture. With headlines like 'eating saturated fat does not cause heart disease' and 'it's the sugar not the fat', people are starting to wonder what they should be eating.[1]

A brief history of fat

To get a better handle on what's going on here, it's probably helpful to dig a little deeper. The complexities are important to unravel, so buckle in.

Saturated fat and cholesterol

The idea that there was a link between lifestyle and heart disease had been knocking around for a while, but it was ultimately consolidated by a groundbreaking study initiated in 1958, called the Seven Countries Study, led by American physiologist Ancel Keys.[2] During this huge research project scientists from across the world worked with Keys to collect and share data, in the hope of identifying links between lifestyle and heart-disease risk. It's important to note that at the time this was a tremendous undertaking. There was no internet, email or home computers. It required the cooperation of scientists from many different countries to work together across the globe. The result, a trilogy of (huge) scientific papers published in 1966, 1970 and 1980, examined data on the lifestyle and rates of heart disease in over 12,700 men from seven countries (the USA, Italy, Finland, Greece, the Netherlands, Japan and what was formerly Yugoslavia), showed a link between the amount of saturated fat (but not total fat) in people's diets and the rate of heart disease.

The complexity of the relationships between what we eat and disease means that nutrition is notoriously hard to study. As such, we need to rely on a range of different study types (which all show us different things) to draw conclusions. In this case, the Seven Countries Study was a very large observational study, which can't show cause and effect, but the findings (increased saturated fat intake is linked to increased heart-disease risk) were backed up by other mechanistic studies, which provided a plausible explanation for this increased risk, namely the impact of saturated fats on blood cholesterol levels.[3]

In addition to this, metabolic ward studies, the most tightly controlled of nutrition study design, as early as the 1950s had shown that saturated fats significantly increased blood cholesterol levels to a greater degree than other fat types. The observations in the Seven Countries Study thus emerged at a time when there was a general understanding of the connection between blood cholesterol (particularly LDL, or low-density lipoprotein) and heart disease. Ultimately, these findings all came together, leading to Ancel Keys proposing the highly influential *diet-heart hypothesis*: the theory that saturated fat raises blood cholesterol levels, which increases your risk of heart disease.

Cholesterol and heart disease

Although it's often viewed as being a harmful substance, cholesterol is an essential component of all our cell walls and is used in some important metabolic functions, such as the production of hormones and vitamin D. It's important! But how is cholesterol linked to heart disease? One thing to note is that when we talk about 'cholesterol', and measure it in the blood, in fact what we're actually measuring are the vehicles that transport cholesterol around the body, which act like wrappers around a sweet. These protein wrappers, known as 'lipoproteins', carry cholesterol around the body to deliver it to cells and to bring it back to the liver when it's been used and needs recycling. We can recognise heart-disease risk by looking at the type of vehicles that our body is using to transport cholesterol around our body; there are certain types of traffic that aren't an issue for our health, and certain types of traffic that are. Heart-disease risk is influenced by the latter.

Something that is often skipped over when discussing cholesterol and heart disease is that cholesterol levels are a 'marker of risk' – not an indication of disease. The development of a complex condition like heart disease is not caused by one single factor, it's influenced, as mentioned before, by our genes, diet, lifestyle, financial and social status, to name just a few. People who have high cholesterol levels may or may not go on to develop heart disease and people have widely varying responses to diet on their cholesterol levels, so a dietary pattern that causes high cholesterol in one person may not do so in another. However, in some people, like those with a genetic condition which predisposes them to high cholesterol (known as familial hypercholesterolemia), the link between high cholesterol and heart disease can be very high.[4] One of the ways cholesterol influences heart-disease risk is that it increases your risk of developing a condition called atherosclerosis. In simple terms, this is the build-up of fatty substances in your arteries, which over time, can narrow your blood vessels and cause a reduced blood flow (and therefore oxygen supply) to your heart muscle. These fatty plaques can also rupture, spilling into your bloodstream, increasing your risk of clots and artery blockages, which could lead to a heart attack or a stroke.

Good and bad cholesterol – how cholesterol affects heart disease risk

Dr Tom Butler PhD, RD, RNutr

Cholesterol is frequently preceded by "good" or "bad" to denote an association with risk of illness. However, when we talk about cholesterol in this context, we are referring to lipoproteins; sphere-like structures that transport cholesterol and fats (triacylglycerols (TAGs)) around the body. However, calling cholesterol "good" or "bad" is a bit oversimplified. Broadly speaking, HDL is considered to be "protective" against heart disease, whereas LDL is a well-established risk factor, but there's a little bit more to it than that.[5]

Although cholesterol metabolism is incredibly complex, in the most basic terms, the structures that transport cholesterol throughout the body (lipoproteins) that we refer to when measuring cholesterol in the blood (and linking to heart-disease risk) have different jobs in this process:

- **Very Low Density Lipoprotein (VLDL):** Made in the liver and takes cholesterol and TAGs from your liver to your body tissues.
- **Low Density Lipoprotein (LDL):** Carries cholesterol to your body's working tissues, for example muscles and other

▶

extra-hepatic tissues, so they can use it (think about this as "outbound" cholesterol transport).

- **High Density Lipoprotein (HDL):** Picks up excess cholesterol in your body after it's been used and takes it back to the liver (consider this "inbound" cholesterol transport).

This is where the idea that high HDL being "good" and LDL being "bad" comes in. The more HDL you have, the more cholesterol can be plucked from the tissues and transported back to the liver for excretion (in theory).

However, these lipoproteins (and the proteins and fats they contain) can be heavily influenced by the environment they are in. For example, a large observational study showed those who had higher levels of an inflammatory marker in their blood and high HDL cholesterol (HDL-C) had an increased risk of death (from all causes, including heart disease). This study and others in this area show us that while a high HDL is a useful marker (and high levels are generally protective), looking at this level alone doesn't tell us everything about your heart-disease risk.[6] Additionally, lower levels of HDL-C have also been linked with lower income, unhealthy lifestyle, higher TAG levels (a blood fat), other cardiac risk factors and diseases. Thus, HDL-C may simply serve as a marker of risk, rather than a risk factor.

The story with LDL is similar. Low levels of LDL cholesterol (LDL-C) are a generally viewed as a good thing for heart health. However, like HDL-C, a low LDL-C alone does not guarantee a low risk of heart disease, it's just one part of the cardiovascular risk puzzle. What is becoming more evident is that additional measures may also be useful to consider alongside the usual

▶

LDL-C and these may help us understand how lipoproteins behave in the body. Such metrics include high blood sugar, high insulin and the presence of insulin resistance. Several studies have also highlighted the value of using other measures, such as non-HDL-C, total cholesterol to high cholesterol ratio (TC:HDL-C), or a fat to cholesterol ratio, known as TAG:HDL-C ratio, all of which may give a more rounded view of risk.[7] [8] [9] On top of all this, there are new areas of research emerging which might fill out our understanding of biomarkers and risk of disease, including the size of the LDL lipoprotein particles that are being measured (known as particle size). This latter point is where a concept of LDL *concordance* and *discordance* comes in. This is very complex, however, in a nutshell it includes the measurement of the amount of cholesterol in LDL (LDL-C), the number of LDL particles, and the size of these particles and seeks to make sense of why some people have a higher prevalence of heart disease but their LDL-C may be relatively normal. It's very complex and we have lots to learn, so watch this space! If we look at what we know right now, having a collective of low HDL-C, high LDL-C, and high TAG altogether appears to be the total picture of a real increase in risk.

How can we pull what seems like quite disparate information together? Is cholesterol implicated in cardiovascular disease? Yes. Is it the biggest and single most important risk factor? Not at all. Hypertension, smoking, insulin resistance are all important risk factors that can modify the amount of cholesterol, the size of particles, the number of particles and ultimately how they function. In an ideal world they all need to be considered when looking at the standard lipid profile. Additionally, improving blood fats through diet and exercise should not be forgotten!

But back to the story. The findings from the Seven Countries Study went on to be echoed by other research, including another large observational study in America, called the Framingham Heart Study (which also highlighted the risks associated with smoking and benefits of exercise in relation to heart disease) and the 1973 NiHonSan Study, which again raised a link between high intakes of saturated fats and heart disease.[10] This was all taking place against a backdrop of growing concern within the US government about rising rates of heart disease.

So what happened? In 1977 the US introduced the first dietary guidelines, the cornerstone of which was advising people to follow a 'low-fat diet', reducing the amount of fat and saturated fats that they ate, with the aim of protecting them from heart disease. In 1983, the UK followed suit, also advising that total fat in the diet be limited to around 30 per cent of energy intake and saturated fat to no more than 10 per cent.[11] This advice led to myriad changes in both our food system (with the proliferation of 'low-fat' foods on the market) and ultimately in the way people ate. It's been suggested that this advice may have directly contributed to a decrease in diet quality for many people, due to promoting an overall belief that if a food is lower in fat it must be healthier.[12]

The state of the controversy

Although absolute numbers of people with heart disease in the UK have fallen since the 90s, it's still a significant problem that affects around seven million people.[13] There has also been a huge spike in the incidence of type 2 diabetes, which, according to statistics from Diabetes UK, has doubled in the past 20 years.[14] This has led to a fierce debate, with some people loudly questioning the links between saturated fat and heart disease found by the Seven Countries Study and the government guidelines that have been shaped by them. More recently, a number of studies that seem to disprove the link between saturated fat and heart disease have been published, leading to further criticism that the longstanding advice to lower fat intake might have inadvertently led to an increase in the intake of refined carbohydrates and driven up rates of type 2 diabetes and heart disease.[15]

One study that has driven this debate is a meta-analysis of observational studies carried out by Siri-Tarino et al in 2010.[16] Unlike Keys, they concluded that saturated fat was not meaningfully linked to an increased risk of heart disease, instead highlighting that the replacement of saturated fats with carbohydrates may be an important factor to consider. Their concerns mimicked those of an earlier study, whereby a large pooled analysis (totalling around 344,000 people) found that replacing saturated fats with carbs increases the risk of having a 'coronary event' (or heart attack).[17] However, they did note the heart health benefits of replacing saturated fats with polyunsaturated fats. So although replacing sources of saturated fat in the diet with sources of refined carbohydrates seems to increase people's risk of heart disease, replacing it with unsaturated fats appears to lower it.

While some of these studies show us that it is important to consider the replacement nutrient when advising people to reduce saturated fat, there are some good reasons why their studies may not have shown a link between saturated fat and heart disease.[18]

Over to our friend, nutritionist and lawyer Alan Flanagan, who sums up the problems with rejecting saturated fat as a marker of risk, based on these studies.

Talking point: measuring the effects of fatty acids on health is tricky (and largely irrelevant)

Alan Flanagan

Many of the recent studies suggesting there is 'no association' between saturated fat and heart disease have been meta-analyses looking at the effects of individual fatty acids (the compounds that fats are made from).

Why might these studies be problematic? Because people don't eat isolated fatts: they eat *foods*. Meta-analyses looking at isolated fatty acids are a manifestation of a recognised issue in nutrition science, that attempting to translate the effect of a *single nutrient* on a *single endpoint* (like LDL cholesterol) into an accurate reflection of the effect of a complex food matrix of other nutrients, and an overall diet pattern, on multifactorial disease processes, is often misleading.

An example of this can be seen in monounsaturated fats, often touted as the 'Mediterranean fats' – olive oil, nuts and avocado. However, meta-analyses of isolated fatty acids would suggest monounsaturated fats might *increase* risk of heart disease! What gives? Well, recall that no food is exclusively one fat type: many foods, such as butter, meats and processed foods, also contain a lot of monounsaturated fats.

What in fact these meta-analyses were reflecting was that at a population level the foods primarily contributing to monounsaturated fat intake were largely animal sources and processed foods, not the plant-sourced fats we associate with cardiovascular health from controlled studies on the Mediterranean diet.

This issue is crucially important and often overlooked when

▶

we arbitrarily discuss 'high' or 'low' anything in the diet: what are the foods providing a particular nutrient, and what is the effect of food in the overall diet pattern? When it comes to an overall diet pattern, and the foods within it, a hierarchy is clear: higher intake of unsaturated fats and complex carbohydrates is more beneficial to health than high intake of saturated fat.

Thus, even if we take the argument for saturated fat at its absolute highest – which is that they're not as bad as we once thought – they are still the *least healthful* option for you.

So, looking at isolated fatty acids, without accounting for the overall diet pattern leads to misleading conclusions. If we look at this issue at the level of food, the pattern is clear: diets rich in unsaturated fats are beneficial to heart health, particularly where they are consumed in a diet pattern with high-fibre, whole grain carbohydrates.

So that's the kicker. People can obsess and argue over the details of the studies and release press statements saying things like 'saturated fats do not clog your arteries', but actually, to us, the people eating the foods, this information is largely irrelevant. What's important for health (from a dietary perspective), as we will discuss in our balance chapter, is which *foods* are on your plate and what sort of foods you choose *most* of the time.

Is dairy fat so scary?

A good example of why labelling foods as good or bad based on levels of one constituent nutrient is unhelpful are dairy foods. Dairy is often a target group when looking to reduce fat in the diet due to the high fat (and saturated fat) content of dairy foods like milk, cheese and yoghurt. The expectation is that the high saturated fat content of these foods will increase blood cholesterol levels, leading to an increased risk of heart disease. However, a recent comprehensive review of the scientific evidence found that eating either full-fat or low-fat dairy foods isn't linked with an increased risk of heart disease.[19] Other studies have also shown that certain types of dairy, like yoghurt and cheese, are linked to a lower incidence of heart disease and type 2 diabetes. This might sound strange, but there is something that scientists think explains these effects: their packaging.

The fats in milk are packed differently to other fats. They come suspended in the liquid part of milk, cased in a complex spherical structure known as the milk fat globule membrane.[20] This membrane is made up of a complex mix of proteins, enzymes and other fats, and it's thought to have an effect on the way we absorb and utilise the fats in milk. Experiments testing this idea have found results that back up this line of thought. For example, a recent study that compared the impact of milk fat either in or out of the milk fat globule membrane found that the fats contained within the structure did not have the same negative effects on the blood levels of study participants.[21]

We don't currently know exactly why this occurs, but it also could explain why different dairy foods have different effects on blood cholesterol levels. Butter, for example (which has fewer fats contained within the milk protein globule membrane), has a greater effect on blood cholesterol than milk or cheese. Overall, these examples are just some of many that show us that foods are more than the sum of their parts – meaning that we can't really judge a food (or its effect on health) based purely on its constituent nutrients.[22]

Myth busting: butter in your coffee and an example of flawed nutrition logic

One nutrition trend that doesn't seem to be going anywhere is 'bulletproof coffee'. For those of you who don't know, Bulletproof coffee is your morning pick-me-up with a little added extra . . . 1–2 tablespoons of butter and 1 tablespoon of MCT oil (Medium Chain Triglycerides, for the science nerds out there) to be exact. Yep. You read that right. Coffee with BUTTER. (And some more fats for good measure.)

Advocates claim that a morning dose of their special blend of 'high-performance' beans plus grass-fed butter and MCTs will do all sorts of magical things, from promoting weight loss to improving brain power. SIGH. So, what's the logic?

Bulletproof coffee was started by Silicon Valley entrepreneur Dave Asprey, a businessman with a special interest in health (note: mostly his own). He first came across yak-butter tea in Tibet and he credits this discovery with his invention of the buttery coffee he swears is a fast track to good health, weight loss and improved focus. Since he is a businessman (not a scientist), who has made a nice profit from his Bulletproof products and trademarked goods, I'm sure we don't need to spell it out that there is a component of money making involved in these claims. However, we'd say part of this product's popularity comes back to the saturated fat debate again, and a large dose of poor nutrition logic.

When the headlines hit, claiming no link had been found between saturated fat and heart disease, our binary thinking kicked in. YES, the nutrition quacks and high-fat-diet lovers

▶

cried! If saturated fat isn't *bad for us*, it MUST be good. The more of it the better! Lather it on your toast, pile it onto your potatoes . . . stick it in your coffee!!

Err. No . . .

Our thoughts

If you replace your usually nutrient-filled breakfast with a Bullet-proof coffee, you're missing out on all the other good stuff that your breakfast could provide you with. Saturated fat may not be the devil we once thought, but that doesn't make it a health food, folks.

How much fat?

Whereas the type of fat certainly seems to be important for heart-disease risk and most experts agree that while we shouldn't be eating high amounts of saturated fat, the total amount of fat in our diet seems to be less important. Indeed, many dietary patterns that are higher in total fat, such as the Mediterranean diet, have been shown to be beneficial for heart health. Experts have also suggested that if we improve our dietary quality as a whole – eating healthy fats, from oily fish and vegetable oils, whole grains, fruits and vegetables – the overall amount of saturated fat in our diets is likely to be less of a concern.[23] And this approach to reducing heart-disease risk would seem to make the most sense. Talking about the percentage of individual saturated fatty acids in our diets is confusing and complex. As previously stated, we don't eat individual nutrients, we eat food, so striving towards making sustainable, healthy changes to our dietary patterns is more actionable and straightforward than trying to manipulate specific nutrients.

So where does this leave us? From a scientific perspective, replacing saturated fat with unsaturated fats is universally agreed to be better for your health. That said, saturated fat is really hard to study, and scientists are increasingly moving away from their focus on single nutrients as a risk for disease and focusing on foods and dietary patterns. We need fats in our diet and certainly don't need to be frightened of them. But instead of worrying about how much saturated fat is in your diet, read on to learn how to choose foods that include healthful fats.

Fats in practice

Food sources of fat are never all saturated or unsaturated; they tend to provide both, just in different proportions. Depending on which combination of three fatty acids are in a fat molecule, the fat in a food might be *mostly* saturated or *mostly* unsaturated. Note we use the word 'mostly'. Butter, for example, is approximately 63 per cent saturated fat, 26 per cent monounsaturated fat and 4 per cent polyunsaturated fat.[24] It's predominantly saturated, so it tends to be dubbed a saturated fat, even though it's not 100 per cent. Olive oil is about 14 per cent saturated, 73 per cent monounsaturated and 8 per cent polyunsaturated fat.[25] As it's mostly unsaturated it tends to be labelled as such.

Generally speaking, an easy way to work out whether a fat contains mostly saturated fats is whether it's liquid or solid at room temperature. A saturated fat such as coconut oil, lard or butter is made up mostly of saturated fatty acids that are solid at room temperature (and gradually turn to liquid if heated up). Unsaturated fats such as olive oil are made up mostly of unsaturated fatty acids, which tend to be liquid or less firm at room temperature. But they can solidify. Have you ever put your olive oil in the fridge? If so, it might have gone waxy, cloudy or even solid. This is because although monounsaturated fats are liquid at room temperature, they will solidify if cooled. Polyunsaturated fats such as sunflower oil or flaxseed oil are made up predominantly of polyunsaturated fatty acids, which are also liquid at room temperature, but they remain in a liquid state if cooled.

Trans fats

Trans fats are the ones that everyone agrees are pretty bad for your health. We know that trans fats are unhealthy because they decrease LDL cholesterol and increase triglycerides in the blood (which is generally considered an unfavourable thing to happen to your blood fats) and they appear to increase the risk for heart disease, too.[26] They should therefore be kept to a minimum, but the good news is that the UK National Food Survey suggests the UK manages to eat within the recommended limits already.[27]

Despite the margarine-haters and their scaremongering, in the UK most manufacturers have significantly reduced the amount of trans fats in their products in recent years. Although there is no law currently requiring food manufacturers to label foods containing trans fats, you can check the ingredients list to see if they contain partially hydrogenated fat/oil or hydrogenated fat/oil (see our food labelling section at the end of the book). The higher up the ingredients list this is, the more trans fats the product is likely to contain. Foods most likely to contain trans fats are those made using hardened vegetables oils, such as biscuits, cakes and pastries.

Talking point: is coconut oil good for me?
Maeve Hanan, registered dietitian at
Dietetically Speaking

Coconut oil is a solid oil that is extracted from the flesh of coco-nuts. It has gained a lot of popularity recently as a superfood with numerous health benefits. There are even dramatic claims that coconut oil can be used to treat medical conditions such as diabetes, irritable bowel syndrome (IBS), Crohn's disease, thyroid disease, Alzheimer's disease, Parkinson's disease, AIDS and cancer.

However, most of these claims are not backed by scientific evidence. Overall, more research is needed to see how coconut oil affects our health, so it is really important to highlight that there is currently no good evidence that coconut oil can be used as a treatment for any medical condition.[28]

One of the most popular claims about coconut oil is that it can promote weight loss by affecting our metabolism and appetite. This is because it contains a type of fat called medium chain triglycerides (MCTs) which have been found to have this effect when given in specific amounts. However, there is no good evidence that coconut oil has the same effect as MCT oil.[29] Lauric acid is the main type of fat in coconut oil, and there is disagreement about whether this is an MCT fat, as it does not have the same effect in our body as other MCTs. Therefore, coconut oil only contains around 23 per cent of the MCTs that act in the same way as MCT oil.[30] Like all types of oil, coconut oil is a high-calorie food. One tablespoon contains about 120 calories, which is roughly the same as half a jam doughnut. So adding a lot of coconut

▶

Fats   47

oil to your diet could cause weight gain as a result of additional calories.

When it comes to heart health, the best available evidence
has found that coconut oil increases cholesterol more than
vegetable oils (such as olive oil and safflower oil), but less than
butter.[31] Coconut oil is also very high in saturated fat, and for
this reason we are advised to only consume it in small amounts
for good heart health. For example, coconut oil contains 82
per cent saturated fat, whereas butter contains 63 per cent
saturated fat and olive oil contains 14 per cent saturated fat.[32]

Coconut oil is also promoted as being a good oil to cook
with as it remains stable when heated. However, this is only
the case with refined coconut oil, whereas the more popular cold-pressed or virgin coconut oil has a medium smoke
point of 180°C, which means that it isn't the best choice
for frying or baking. Healthier oils, such as refined olive oil,
rapeseed oil and avocado oil are better choices for high-
temperature cooking.

If you enjoy the taste of coconut oil it is fine to include it in
small amounts as part of a balanced diet. However, there is
currently no good evidence that it has any miraculous health
benefits. Unless you are trying to increase your calorie intake,
there is no need to add it to your coffee or indeed elsewhere
for its health benefits!

So what fats should we be eating?

To promote good health, the general rule of thumb is to try
to get most of your fat from unsaturated sources. This doesn't
mean that you should never eat foods you enjoy that are high in

saturated fat (you don't need to be all or nothing!), just choose those that are higher in unsaturated fats as your main sources, most of the time. This means including sources of healthy fats in your diet, like oily fish (aim for at least one portion a week), choosing nuts as a snack and cooking with unsaturated oils (such as rapeseed or olive). A top tip is that that rapeseed (or canola) oil is often labelled as vegetable oil in the UK, making it an affordable oil to use in cooking. All advice stands, whatever the macronutrient content of your diet is. So if your diet is low in fat, try to ensure you're not replacing fats with refined carbohydrates, and even if you choose to follow a diet lower in carbohydrates and higher in fats, try ensuring you get most of your fats from unsaturated sources – simple.

Sources of (mostly) unsaturated fats

Avocado
Olives
Oils (sesame, olive, rapeseed/canola, peanut)
Seeds (sesame)
Oily fish
Marine algae
Nuts, e.g. walnuts and pine nuts
Seeds, e.g. pumpkin seeds, flaxseeds, chia seeds and sunflower seeds
Fortified eggs

Oily fish – what counts?
Anchovies
Carp
Herring (including kipper)
Mackerel
Pilchards
Salmon
Sardines
Trout
Whitebait

4

Carbohydrates

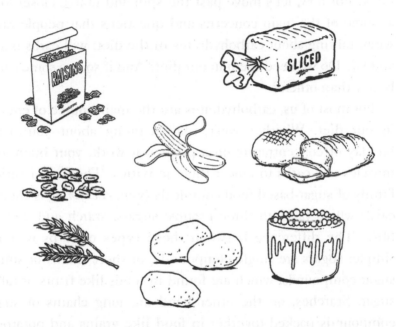

Carbs are currently top of the list of nutrients we love to hate. To us, it's unsurprising that most people have a love-hate relationship with them. They are tasty and filling, but as a nutrient they are plagued by controversy and are often the subject of confusion. We're told they're the root of all our dietary ills: toxic, fattening and addictive. They have been blamed for the rise of all sorts of public health problems, from diabetes to heart disease and even cancer.[1][2] Recent media hype saw two studies with almost identical findings (that getting around half your energy from carbs was associated with the lowest risk of death) generating headlines with opposite claims. The first study led to reports that low-carb diets were the healthiest, the other led to headlines stating it could lower your life expectancy by five years! But don't fear, despite the media hype and their terrible reputation, focusing on a single macronutrient (like carbs) as the cause of poor health isn't really helpful (or scientific), the reasons for which we will explain later in this book. For now, let's move past the spin and take a closer look at some of the main concerns and questions that people raise when talking about carbohydrates in the diet: will carbs make you fat? Do we need them in our diet? And if so, are some carbs better than others?

For most of us, carbohydrates are the main source of energy in our diet. Whether you're daydreaming about your next holiday or concentrating on a project at work, your brain and muscles use carbs to power their activities. They are a varied family of sugar-based food chemicals (yup, *everything* is chemicals!) which fall into three groups: sugars, starch and dietary fibre. The difference between these types of carbs is quite simple: sugars are single compounds, or short chains of single sugar compounds, which are found in foods like fruits or table sugar. Starches, on the other hand are long chains of sugar compounds packed together in food like grains and potatoes. And finally, fibre is a form of non-digestible carbohydrate – long chains of sugars that pass through our gut undigested, as we can't break them down (roughage, if you will). Apart from the sugar found in milk, carbohydrates pretty much only come from plants, which you might know use sunlight to create sugar (via a process called photosynthesis), which can further be converted to starch and fibre. Yup. Plants. That doesn't sound so scary does it? So why the controversy?

Will carbs make me fat?

The most common concern we hear about carbohydrates is that they are uniquely fattening, so should be avoided by people who want to lose weight or prevent weight gain. How many times have you heard that to lose weight you should 'cut the carbs'? Confusingly, there are mixed opinions shared about this from health professionals and scientists in the media. Some health professionals loudly agree with this statement and promote low-carb diets as the solution to the nation's weight and health problems, and others dispute this, saying it's a confusing and misleading statement. This is coupled with a large number of vocal people who feel let down by government advice, people who switched to a low-carb diet and found it helped them. Who's right? (Spoiler alert: there isn't a simple, one-size-fits-all answer.) Let's roll back to the science to explain.

The belief that carbs are uniquely fattening comes from a theory in nutrition science called the 'carbohydrate-insulin hypothesis' (hypothesis just being a fancy word for theory). This theory suggests that carbohydrates drive weight gain through their effects on one of our body's hormones, insulin.

Quick recap: like other hormones, insulin is a chemical messenger that works in our body to control bodily functions; in this case, one of insulin's main jobs is to regulate our blood sugar levels. In simple terms, when we eat carbohydrate-containing foods, our blood sugar goes up and our pancreas responds by releasing insulin. This does two things; firstly, it tells our body to move sugar (glucose) from our blood into our cells and increase storage of fat. Secondly, it prevents the breakdown of stored fats and proteins for energy – so we 'burn' sugars for fuel.

This theory kind of makes sense, right? Eating carbs means insulin levels go up, so we break down less fat and move more of it into storage. Therefore, the line of thought goes, carbohydrates are more fattening than other nutrients and people who follow a lower-carbohydrate diet will lower their insulin levels and burn more fat than people who eat carbs. Simple.

But wait! That's not exactly what the science says.

One way to test this theory would be to measure the macro-nutrient content of people's diets to determine if lower amounts of carbs (and lower insulin levels) lead to greater weight loss, even when people were eating the same amount of calories. Testing this in the real world is hard; people are notoriously bad at knowing what they are eating, which means it's difficult to know how many carbs/how much fat is in a person's diet, even if they say they know. To accurately measure the effects of different nutrients in a controlled way, scientists carry out what are known as 'metabolic ward studies', where the participants in the science trial live in a controlled environment. Every last bit of movement and food intake is measured and recorded. In other words, there's no 'cheating' or misreporting: these studies are highly accurate.

If high levels of insulin in our blood (caused by carbohydrates in the diet) promotes fat gain (as per carb-insulin hypothesis), lowering the carb content of the diet should decrease insulin levels and promote more fat loss. This means that in metabolic ward studies those eating the same amount of calories from a higher-carb diet will lose less weight than those on the low-carb diet. However, we know from these studies that that's not the case. Many metabolic ward studies have shown that (when calories and protein are kept the same) the percentage of dietary fat or carbohydrate in a diet makes very little difference to the amount of weight lost. In fact, a recent meta-analysis (which systematically reviewed studies that looked at this) confirmed that the amount of carbs or fat has little to do with the amount of fat burned, despite differences in the amount of insulin people had circulating in their bodies.[3]

But what about weight *gain*, we hear you cry? Nope. Carbs don't make you gain more weight than fat either.

To see the effects on weight gain, we can look at what are called 'overfeeding studies'. These clinical trials do exactly what they say on the tin: feed people more calories than they need, so we can monitor the effects. Overfeeding studies have found that both overfeeding carbs and fat cause an increase in weight, and that there is little difference between the two macronutrients.[4]

So why is this? Well, it's because in these studies calories were matched and, ultimately, when it comes down to it, it's calories (rather than nutrients) that make a difference to weight. However, again, this is only part of the story! In the real world, only looking at nutrients or calories also misses the complexity of the discussion about weight. Energy balance (and therefore body weight) is determined by a vast number of interactions between biological, psychological and social factors, some of which are under individual control (and many of which are not) that make weight (and weight loss) unimaginably complex.[5]

Low-carb diets

Low-carbohydrate diets are increasingly popular, with lots of people now opting to cut carbs from their diets with the hope of losing weight or improving their health. In fact, if people want to lose weight, one of the first (well-meaning) nuggets of advice often offered is to cut carbs, probably because most people think that carbs are inherently 'fattening'. However, before we get into that, let's explore what we really mean when we talk 'low carb'.

Often referred to as a single entity, low-carb diets can look quite different. What they all have in common is that they involve restricting the amount of total carbohydrates in your diet. However, the amount you actually restrict can vary. Many people make the unconscious leap from 'reducing carbs might be good for some people' to 'all carbs are evil and toxic', leading them to thinking that 'low-carb' means 'no carbs', which is a very different thing. You don't have to be ketogenic or following the recently popular, all-meat 'carnivore' lifestyle to be following a low- (or lower-) carb diet!

So what is a low-carb diet?

Low-carb diets recommend eating foods like meats, fish, chicken, eggs, nuts, seeds and high-fat dairy, as well as fruits and vegetables. Some reduced (but moderate) carb diets even include small amounts of carbohydrate-heavy foods such as root vegetables, potatoes and grains.

Types of low-carb diets

Interestingly, despite all the hype there is no universally agreed definition of low-carb diets. In studies, they are usually defined as per centages of diets (with >45 per cent generally being considered high carb and <26 per cent being low). In a practical sense, though, the following sums up how many people categorise the diets:

Category	Max carb intake per day	Example diets
Moderate carb	130–225 grams	Mediterranean (PREDIMED)
Low-carb	<103 grams	South Beach
Very low-carb (ketogenic)	<50 grams	ketogenic diet Atkins

Quite often these diets also have a focus on eating 'whole' or minimally processed foods; although it's perfectly possible to find low-carb convenience food these days, one of the most important things to realise about people who switch over to this dietary pattern is that they may experience quite a shift in their eating habits and the 'quality' of their overall diet.

Why do some people recommend a low-carb diet?

It's not the carbs that are fattening, per se, but aren't there other reasons why a diet lower in carbohydrates may be helpful? Common reasons why some people promote these diets are because they claim they feel less hungry, they lose weight quicker and they find them easier to maintain.

Hunger

Often people who prefer or promote low-carb diets state that they make them feel less hungry. People who eat lower-carb diets often end up eating more protein, which *may* make them feel fuller and result in them eating fewer calories, without them really noticing.[6] That said, appetite is influenced by many different factors including emotions, environment and activity (to name just a few) so eating less on a low-carb diet certainly isn't a guarantee.

Faster short-term weight loss

One reason why some people love following low-carb diets for weight loss is that they initially appear to work better. In the short term this is true and many people lose weight quickly in the initial stages of the diet, which is less to do with fat-burning efficiency and more to do with a loss of water weight.[7] Rapid reductions in weight in the initial stages of a low-carb diet are due to the carb stores in your muscles (glycogen) being depleted.[8] Glycogen is stored with water, so as you use it up, you lose some 'water weight' along with it, giving the illusion of fast fat loss.

After about 12 months, however, on average there is no difference between low-carb and low-fat diets for weight loss.[9] Like any diet, the results were also very variable between people. Some people lost weight, others gained weight and some stayed around the same. However, although it's not often mentioned when talking about weight, most people who go on a diet will regain the weight they have lost in the long term.[10]

An automatic reduction in high-fat, high-sugar foods in your diet

Choosing to eat low-carb may mean a huge shift in eating patterns. This automatically rules out lots of foods that can contribute large amounts of calories to your daily diet. These foods include staple carbohydrates such as bread, pasta, rice and potatoes, but perhaps more importantly, things like cakes, biscuits and other high-fat, high-sugar snack foods. This simple shift can cause a vast change to your dietary pattern and marked improvements in your dietary quality, because these foods aren't on the menu so often.

But what do studies of a low-carb diet say?

Overall, long-term studies which have looked at low-carb versus low-fat diets in the 'real world' outside the rigorous testing of metabolic wards have all found the same thing: that on average, there's no difference in the effectiveness of low-carb and low-fat diets for weight loss in the longer term.

The most recent (and quite possibly best) example of this was the landmark DIETFITS study, a huge, high-quality, randomised controlled trial which pitted low-carb diet against a low-fat diet in over 600 people over a 12-month period.[11] The participant group for this study (middle-aged adults with no pre-existing health conditions and a BMI between 30 and 39.9) were randomly assigned to either a low-carb or a low-fat diet for the 12-month period. During this time, they had their intake carefully monitored to see how well they stuck to the diet they were prescribed. This was important, as participants were told to keep to very low-carb or low-fat for the first two months, then increase their intake of these nutrients to the minimum level that they could tolerate for the duration of the year. Even more interestingly, participants were also looked at to see if either insulin resistance or their genes could explain whether they were successful at losing weight. Everyone was well supported throughout the trial, offered regular dietitian counselling and encouraged to follow a high-quality 'whole foods' diet.

So what happened?

Overall, there was no difference in weight loss between the low-fat and low-carb groups and successful weight loss could not be explained by people's genetic characteristics or circulating insulin levels. Neither group stuck to the very low levels of carbs or fat in their diet as the diet progressed – this often happens with nutrient prescriptions, which are very difficult to stick to in real life. Both groups saw positive changes to health markers such as cholesterol levels, blood pressure, waist circumference and fasting insulin levels.

Most noticeably, as expected, there was huge individual variability in people's responses to the diet, which means that even though on average there is no difference between the groups, some people lost lots of weight and others gained (in both groups).

However, all this aside, it's also important to remember that although diets are popular for weight loss and success in the short term is possible, over the long term most people regain the weight they have lost on a diet (and many end up heavier than they were before).[12] So, while following a low-carb lifestyle may suit you (and for some, particularly people with diabetes, help you control your health condition), there is no one 'best' dietary pattern for everyone. The best one for you is one that meets your needs, that you enjoy and that you can follow in the long term.

Carbs aren't an essential nutrient

One of the most common things people who advocate for a low-carb diet will say when giving their reasoning for minimising carbohydrate intake (or trying to convince you to) is that carbs aren't an essential nutrient and we can get on just fine without them. More than this, some people think that because carbs aren't essential, they must be toxic!

What's the truth?

It's true that carbs are not essential to your survival, and by this we mean that if you don't eat them (but are eating enough calories from fat and protein), your body can use the protein and fat to create ketone bodies and glucose, so you won't die. BUT don't mistake 'not essential' with 'not beneficial'. Not dying is hardly a glowing review of anything. In fact, some evolutionary scientists have linked carbohydrate with the evolution of the large modern human brain, indicating that its inclusion in our diet could be linked with the accelerated growth and development of the human race.[13]

Certainly, when you're talking about health benefits of carbs, quality counts. We know that 'quality' carbs such as whole grains, fruits and vegetables have been linked with all sorts of health benefits, from improving your gut health to reducing your risk of disease. This argument against carbs just doesn't stack up.

Low-carb or high-carb diets for health?

This is the impossible question to answer that still leads people into heated arguments about 'the best diet'. Annoyingly, although it would solve a lot of problems (and save many keyboard warriors a few hours of arguing on Twitter every day), we can't answer this question with absolutes. To demonstrate this, let's take a look at the two studies that we mentioned right at the start, the ones that both found that getting around half your energy intake from carbs was probably optimum, but ended up being held up in arguments about low-carb (e.g. low-carb/high-fat diets) and high-carb (e.g. veganism) as 'proof' that one way of eating was better than another.[14] The two studies in question are PURE (which stands for Prospective Urban and Rural Epidemiological Study, or in English: following and studying what people in different countries ate for a bit) and ARIC (which is an acronym for Atherosclerosis Risk in Communities – scientists love an acronym!). Although the overall data from these studies pointed to a moderate carb intake being linked with the lowest risk of disease and dying during the study period, headlines like 'Low-fat diets could kill you' and 'Low-carb diets could shorten life' dominated the press, making it seem as though they found completely different things and contradicted each other.[15] [16] There were many differences in the way these studies were carried out, PURE looked at the eating habits of around 135,000 people in 18 countries over 10 years, where ARIC studied just over 15,000 people in the US for 25 years. Both are observational studies, which means they can't tell us if carb intake causes more (or less) death and disease, but they can show trends and patterns. It's probably worth mentioning at this point that they weren't studying high versus low carb as absolute or standard measurements – they classified diets as high or low in carbohydrate in relative terms, based on what people said they were eating. In PURE, 'low-carb' was around 46 per cent of energy from carbs and in ARIC any intake less than 40 per cent, which is still pretty high ...

What did these studies *actually* tell us?

The food we eat is a complex combination of not just macronutrients like carbs and fats, but different food choices and nutrients, all tied up with complex genetic, social and environmental factors – such as how much money we have and whether we have good access to food and healthcare (to name the tiniest, tiniest number of things in the much bigger picture). These two studies, like many before them, amongst other things added to the evidence that, in general, having access to a variety of foods and getting a balance of nutrients is important for your health.

So, top tip, when you see a headline claiming one dietary pattern is better than another, you can just skip that one and keep on keeping on with your day. You're welcome.

What happens if we don't eat enough carbohydrates?

Our brain, nerve cells and red blood cells prefer to use glucose as their main source of fuel. If there is not enough glucose in the blood from the diet, the body is forced to use fats and protein to keep these important bodily functions running. This situation can occur in starvation, where (as mentioned) an inadequate supply of calories and carbs in the diet shifts the way fats are usually metabolised to produce energy, in the form of ketone bodies. However, our bodies can also be tricked into ketosis by consuming a low-carb, low(ish) protein and high-fat diet called a ketogenic diet, which we discuss in the popular diets section, later on.

Carbs in practice

The actual amount of carbohydrate you need to eat will depend on your individual needs; or, more crudely, how active you are and what your dietary pattern of choice is. For example, if you work at a desk and have a sedentary job, you probably don't need as much as a person who works on a building site or who is active all day long. Likewise, people who follow a dietary pattern like veganism will need to eat more carbs to meet their needs than somebody who has chosen to follow a diet which is carb-restricted. Both dietary patterns can be healthy, even though they contain different proportions of carbohydrates.

When you eat carbs: think quality (most of the time)

If you've heard carbs are 'bad' for you, think again. Some are healthier than others (tragically, eating cola bottles all day is not excellent for your physical health). But when eating carbs, the type you choose can really make a positive impact on your health. It's the quality that counts! Lower-quality carbs tend to include refined grains such as white bread, white rice, pastries, confectionery and sweetened drinks. High-quality carbs tend to come from fruits, vegetables, whole grains, beans and legumes. The 'wholeness' and fibre content of these foods are what makes them healthier. That's not to say you can't ever eat refined grains (sometimes the 'healthiest' choice isn't the most nutritious!) – just from a health perspective, whole grains are better, so we should go for these *most* of the time. So why is this?

Carbs = fibre

Although we focus a lot on the suggested negative effects of carbs, talking about them as a pure energy source and not much else, we rarely shout about their benefits. One of these is that carb-containing foods are often where we find fibre, and fibre is considered pretty good for us. Researchers have estimated that every 7 grams extra of fibre per day (that's a half can portion of baked beans) is linked with a 9 per cent reduction in heart disease, 7 per cent reduction in strokes and 8 per cent reduction in colorectal cancer.[17] Recommendations were made in 2014 to increase the population's daily target from 18 grams per day to 30. However, as a nation we're eating much less than this, with an average intake of around 18 grams per day, meaning most of us are falling short by about 40 per cent.[18]

Although from an academic perspective, definitions and categories of fibre can change, it's historically been divided into two groups based on how it behaves in the body: soluble fibre, found in foods like oats and fruit, dissolves in water forming a sticky gel which helps you to form nice soft poos (no straining on the loo!) and it's also easily digested (aka fermented) by bacteria in the colon, so it supports good gut health. Including this type of fibre in your diet may also help you maintain good blood sugar control and healthy cholesterol levels – so it's very multifunctional! Insoluble fibre found in foods like whole grains and nuts doesn't dissolve in water and is difficult for your gut bacteria to digest. This fibre, however, adds bulk to your poo, making it heavy and firm and easier to pass (#poochat).

Fibre-rich foods

- Fruit.
- Vegetables.
- Nuts.
- Seeds.
- Peas, beans and pulses.
- Potatoes with their skin.

How to increase fibre in your diet

- Choose a high-fibre, whole-grain breakfast cereal (aim for at least 6 grams fibre per 100 grams).
- Add fruit (including dried) and/or nuts and seeds to cereal or yoghurt. This could include linseeds.
- Choose a whole grain loaf of bread (see below how to do this).
- Keep your freezer well-stocked with frozen fruit (such as berries) and veg.
- Choose wholemeal pasta.
- Snack on fruit (including dried), nuts, oatcakes, crudites and hummus.
- Add beans, peas, pulses and veggies to pasta, stews, Bolognese, sauces, salads and side dishes.
- After washing, leave the skin on fruit and vegetables.
- It's important to go slow if you're increasing the fibre in your diet. Do this gradually to avoid any tummy troubles such as bloating and gas to give your gut time to adjust. Drink enough fluids, too, to help the fibre work its magic effectively.

Why should we choose whole grains?

You've probably heard people (including us, two paragraphs up in this book) natter on about whole grains as examples of quality carbohydrates, but what are they?

Plant-wise, grains are the edible seeds of cereal crops such as wheat, rye, oats, rice and barley (however, we often class seeds such as amaranth, buckwheat, quinoa and wild rice as grains as well, even though they grow on a different group of plants). But, despite knowing where they come from, there's no unifying definition for whole grains that has been agreed globally (which is part of the problem). An EU-funded project called HEALTHGRAIN has attempted to resolve this and it has come up with a very logical definition, which explicitly states that 'whole grains' should quite literally contain the *whole grain:* the rich outer bran, the germ (a nutrient-packed inner layer) and the endosperm (the grain's starchy innards).[19] Refined grains, however, (think white flour or white bread) have had the fibrous bran and nutritious germ layer removed during processing, leaving only the starchy endosperm. This means whole grains can contain up to 75 per cent more nutrients compared to refined cereals.

Examples of whole grains and pseudo-cereals

Whole grains

- Rice (brown, black, red, wild).
- Wild rice (not technically from a cereal grass).
- Wheat (spelt and durum).
- Barley (not pearled).
- Maize (corn).
- Rye (oats).

- Teff.
- Sorghum.

Pseudo-cereals
- Buckwheat.
- Quinoa.
- Kamut.
- Freekeh.
- Millet.
- Amaranth.

From a science standpoint, the evidence suggests that whole grains are a healthy choice, linking them with a reduced risk of heart disease and diabetes, weight gain and even premature death.[20] In fact, a recent meta-analysis pooling 12 different science studies found that people who ate 70 grams of whole grains per day (about four servings), compared to those who ate very little were about 20 per cent less likely to die during the trial.[21] It's the wholeness of whole grains – the fact that they contain many beneficial nutrients, including phytochemicals (plant nutrients), good fats, fibre (compared to refined grains), which is thought to be the reason for their healthiness. Refined carbohydrate foods have often had many of these removed, before being combined with added sugars and saturated fats, making them distinctly lacking in fibre in comparison. Some of the fibre in whole grains also helps to move food quicker along the digestive tract, reducing the time during which potentially damaging substances are in contact with the gut wall. Other fibres can feed the good bacteria, too, helping them to increase the production of substances (such as special fats called short-chain fatty acids) which keep the gut wall healthy.

BUT we need to make more of an effort to swap from refined

to whole grains. Surveys show about 95 per cent of us don't get enough and one in three of us don't get any at all![22]

What's interesting is that many people think they know what whole grain means, but are being duped by clever flowery language on food labels referring to 'wholeness'. Terms like 'seeded', 'multigrain' or 'wholesome' may sound like that food is healthy (and whole grain!), but these words are often nothing more than misleading phrases, trying to 'health-up' a refined grain product. What's more, whilst the terms 'high-fibre' and 'wholemeal' are legally protected, 'whole grain' isn't and has become a bit of a buzzword! And the fact that some of the products we're buying may not contain all the whole grain goodness we're expecting, makes it extremely difficult for us shoppers to make informed choices.

So how do we know if a food is whole grain? If you're eating grains on their own, such as oats or brown rice, the answer to this is self-explanatory. Or if your bread is made from 100 per cent whole-grain flour, this would be a whole-grain food, too (you'd know this if it said 100 per cent whole-wheat flour on your bread, for example). However, what's not clear is when a packet of food can be called 'whole grain' when it includes refined grains, too.

Whilst in Norway 100 per cent of the flour must be whole grain for it to be labelled 100 per cent whole-grain, in Sweden for a food to be labelled whole grain, at least 50 per cent of the dry ingredients need to be of whole-grain origin, and in the US, whole-grain foods must contain at least 51 per cent whole grain ingredients by weight. In the UK, we have zilch! All that exists is the recommendation for products to contain at least 8 grams of whole grains per portion. BUT this guidance is only voluntary, not legally binding. So this means that when you see a loaf of bread labelled 'whole grain', it might only contain a mere pinch of whole-grain flour as well as containing more added sugar, salt and less healthy fats compared to wholemeal (products made from finely milled wholegrain).

So where does this leave us consumers? Pretty confused, we hear you say! Until there is a legal definition of the term 'whole grain', or the term is banned, it's worth making a special effort to ensure any grains you include in your diet are, quite literally, in their whole form, to get the maximum benefit. You can also try to make sure the first item on the ingredients list includes the word 'whole' (e.g. whole-wheat flour). But there may be a better trick up our sleeve to recognising a wholly whole-grain food; you'll need a teeny bit of maths (or the calculator on your phone) and a food label, but then you're all set.

Bring in the carb to fibre ratio

The ratio of carbohydrates to fibre in a genuine whole grain is approximately 10 grams of carbohydrate for every gram of fibre. Some scientists have recognised that this ratio when applied to whole-grain foods is a good method of identifying foods with more fibre, less sugar and salt. In other words, the ratio can help to work out if your carb is of good quality and as near to a whole grain as possible. Don't let yourself become fanatical about this, but when you're next shopping, have a go.[23]

How to test the wholeness of your whole-grain foods

1) Look at the food label (either per 100 grams or per portion). Multiply the grams of fibre by 10. What number did you get?
2) You are aiming for this number to be larger than the grams of total carbohydrates. This signals that you've got a healthful whole-grain food.

Let's take a well-known branded loaf we found in a supermarket as an example. This loaf has 1.5g of fibre and 9.2g of total carbohydrates per slice.

1) Multiply 1.5g of fibre by 10 = 15.
2) 15 is larger than the carbohydrate figure (9.2g), implying this
    is a pretty 'whole' loaf.

If you include grains in your diet, here's a summary of tips
for choosing whole grains:

• Keep in mind that the term whole grain has not been legally
  defined, and your whole-grain-labelled food may not be as
  healthful as it seems.
• Flowery words such as wholesome, enriched and seeded do
  not guarantee a whole-grain product either.
• Include intact grains and pseudo-cereals in your diet.
• Aim for whole-grain flour to be first or one of the first few on
  the ingredients list.
• Use the 10-to-1 carbohydrate versus fibre ratio when shopping
  for whole-grain food products.

5

Sugar

Yes, yes, we know sugar is a carb, but due to its recent promotion to public health enemy number one, we thought it deserved a chapter in its own right. Previous chart-toppers include fat and salt, but now, with its reputation for bulking out our diets with empty calories and claims that it causes diseases like diabetes and cancer, sugar is officially top of our shit list. The moral panic about the use of sugar in our food has led to media headlines touting it as addictive and toxic. It's led to the diet fans amongst us to 'quit sugar' in our thousands, (usually in the form of switching out table sugar for the 'natural' unrefined alternatives such as honey, coconut syrup and date syrup, which are promoted as healthy, wholesome alternatives by the wellness crowd). But it's not just media hysteria or fringe wellness that has a problem with sugar. Public health messages are riddled with tips for spotting hidden sugars in our food. Parents have been warned that kids in the UK are eating up to twice as much sugar than is recommended[1] and there's a whole host of government-backed apps, lobbyist groups and public health campaigns dedicated to getting us to reduce the stuff in our diets.[2] [3] So what's the deal? Is all sugar bad for us? Should we be switching the white stuff for 'healthier' alternatives? Or using artificial sweeteners instead of sugar? And what about the crowd that's sticking up two fingers to what was previously known as 'clean eating' and having their cake and eating it?! All of these questions make the topic of sugar both an emotionally charged and confusing topic of conversation. But don't worry. We've got you.

Let's start at the beginning.

Like saturated fat, sugar first came to our attention in the 1960s. At this point, nutrition science was still very young (fun fact: the first vitamin wasn't identified until 1926). But this shiny new field, with a track record of successfully tackling deficiency-related conditions, such as rickets and scurvy, now turned its attention to some of the other major health problems of the time, namely heart disease and cancer. During this novel era of nutrition science, we liked to think about food and health in a reductionist manner, focusing on single nutrients in foods as a potential problem, rather than assessing dietary patterns as a whole.[4] At around the same time that Ancel Keys was pushing the theory that saturated fat was linked to heart disease, another scientist, John Yudkin, published an observational study that linked higher sugar consumption to higher rates of heart disease. Although his idea was novel (and thought by many to hold merit), his evidence was not considered quite as compelling as that produced by Keys. This led to other scientists, who were invested in the 'fat causes heart disease' narrative, publicly (and some would say fiercely) opposed to his ideas, favouring the idea that it was fat, not sugar, that was the problem. Undeterred, Yudkin went on to write a book based on his research, called *Pure, White and Deadly*, which highlighted the potential harms of sugar (and sounds a lot like it could sell well in today's sugar-phobic, wellness scene!), but which at the time led to him being largely ostracised by his peers, leaving his career and his ideas in tatters.[5]

So Yudkin was the original proponent of the dangers of sugar, but since then other scientists, (most notably Robert Lustig, as well as journalists like Gary Taubes) have taken this idea and run with it, championing the carbohydrate-insulin model of obesity that we discussed in the 'Carbs' chapter. But 'carbohydrates' encompasses a wide range of foods, including fruits, vegetables, whole grains, cakes and confectionery, as well as other starchy foods, so are they all the same?

Is all sugar equal?

Although we often talk about sugar as though it's one singular entity, it's not. As well as all the different forms in which sugar comes (glucose, sucrose and fructose, for example) it also comes packaged in different ways, such as an apple versus a can of Coke. The sugars that everyone agrees that we should all be eating less of in our diet (as a whole) are what are known as 'free sugars'. (Spoiler alert: this isn't diet language for 'eat it freely', but the name makes sense once you know what it means, honest.[6])

All this considered, how many times have you heard that fruit is 'bad for you' because of the sugar it contains? Or as a recent well-known doctor claimed, that eating starchy foods (e.g. rice or potatoes) was just like 'mainlining sugar', and the current Facebook meme favourite: 'how many teaspoons of sugar are in [insert food here]?' (eyeroll). It's true that if you looked at compounds of sugar found in fruit or starch under a microscope, they would have exactly the same chemical structure, whether they're found in an apple, some chocolate or a sweet potato. So, considering the compounds alone, our body will perceive all of these sugars in the same way, as fuel. However, in the real world, thinking of them in this way doesn't give us the full picture. Despite containing sugar, foods like fruits and vegetables are considered a whole and healthy addition to your diet because the sugars in them are contained inside the cell structure of the food and

because they also contain a range of other nutrients, such as vitamins, minerals and fibre. There's a ton of observational research
that supports this view, linking the consumption of a variety of
sugar containing fruit and veg with health. There's also very limited evidence to support the idea that the natural sugars found
intact within these whole-foods are harmful, even for people who
have problems processing sugars, like those with diabetes.[7] [8]

What are free sugars exactly?

Free sugars are sugars that are no longer found within the cell
wall of the plant that they came from. These are sugars that are
added to food and drinks by cooks, manufacturers and by you in
your cooking and food production at home. If you think about
them as 'added sugars', it can make a bit more sense. As well as
the obvious table sugar, free sugars are also found naturally in
honey and syrups. In the UK, we get most of our free sugars from
table sugar, sugar-sweetened beverages (such as fizzy drinks,
energy drinks, squashes and cordials), as well as cakes, sugar-
sweetened cereals and cereal products (such as breakfast bars).[9]
Although we also consume sugars that are naturally present in
fruit, vegetables, whole grains, milk and milk products such as
natural yoghurt and cheese, these don't count as free sugars. A
yoghurt, for example, would only contain free sugars if sugar has
been added during manufacturing (you could spot this by looking
at the ingredients list for added sugars, purées, syrups or juices).

But what about smoothies and juices? They don't have
added sugar, so are they sugar-free? Not exactly. Fruit juices
and smoothies are often sold as health elixirs, rather than the
fruit-based meal or snack they are, so it comes as a surprise to
many that although their smoothie or juice might contain loads
of fruit, it can only ever count as one portion of their fruit or veg
each day. The same goes if you have a glass of fruit juice, then a
smoothie later. Still just one. But why? The main reason for this
is that these foods can have a relatively high free-sugar content.

When fruit is blended or juiced, the sugars are released from their cells and they become free sugars. Shop-bought smoothies are also often sifted (removing the fibre) to make them smooth and some have additional fruit juice added, too. This means the smoothie in the bottle, while likely to contain vitamins and minerals, is not the same as consuming whole fruit. This doesn't make them unhealthy, though – that sort of good/bad dichotomy doesn't work for food, they just aren't a silver bullet to good health (no matter what the juice dieters say!). The best way to think of it is this: eating fruits has been linked with some health benefits, whole is best (smoothies and juices can count), and unless you have a medical reason to avoid it (like an allergy), you don't need to worry about including it in your diet.

So it's free sugars that we need to be mindful of. But looping back, was Yudkin right? Should we have all been limiting free sugars rather than fat in order to protect ourselves from disease? The answer is (unsatisfyingly) that Yudkin and Keys were both a little bit right, and a little bit wrong. And it's all because they were looking at the same problem from a slightly different (reductionist) perspective.

Let us elaborate.

One of the main things people are currently concerned about when it comes to sugar and health is diabetes. The first thing we should stress, and probably the most important point to make when considering a question like this, is this: diabetes, like other diseases, is not caused by a single food or nutrient. Risk factors for noncommunicable diseases (often misleadingly called 'lifestyle' diseases) include a range of factors, some within and some outside of our control. These include your genes, your environmental and social situation (e.g. your access to food, income, education and housing), as well as your age, ethnicity/race, diet and how stressed and physically active you are (to name just a few). So it's definitely not a one-man show.[10] [11]

WHAT ARE FREE SUGARS?

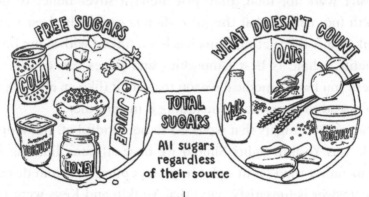

FREE SUGARS

WHAT DOESN'T COUNT

TOTAL SUGARS

All sugars regardless of their source

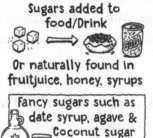

Sugars added to food/Drink

Or naturally found in fruitjuice, honey, syrups

Fancy sugars such as date syrup, agave & Coconut sugar all count too!

Sugars contained naturally within the cell structure of wholefoods, milk and milk products

However, some observational research has linked dietary patterns that are rich in 'free sugars' to disease risk (especially when consumed in liquid form, like fizzy drinks). It's been suggested that this link may be due to sugary drinks being really easy to consume in high amounts (as they don't fill you up) and that consuming lots of sugar in this form may lead to a regular calorie intake that is surplus to your needs. This is thought to be particularly important in diabetes risk, because people who have lots of fat stored inside their abdomen and organs are at a higher risk of developing type 2 diabetes and other diseases (important note: the amount of fat you have stored around your internal organs isn't reliably indicated by weight or BMI, and type 2 diabetes is seen in people of all different body sizes).[12] [13] [14] Looking at sugar specifically, a small number of studies have linked excessive free-sugar consumption to a *higher risk* of depositing fat around the organs[15]. However, the amount of excess sugar people were consuming in these trials was very high. In particular, one study that assigned its participants to drink 1 litre of sugar-sweetened fizzy drinks per day over a six-month period found that they deposited higher amounts of ectopic fat (fat inside organs) than people who drank the same number of calories from milk, water or diet cola.[16] Drinking a litre of Coke per day probably isn't good for you – we're yet to meet anyone who finds this surprising! But does this mean you should never have sugar? That a diet free from fruit juices, cake or a can of Coke will protect you against all ills? Nope.[17] There's a link, but it's a tenuous one, between sugar and the development of diabetes, especially as drinking high numbers of sugary drinks is also linked with less-healthy dietary patterns and with poverty, both of which are risk factors for diabetes.[18] [19] [20]

Although most of the evidence points to consuming high amounts of free sugar being harmful, eating some foods high in free sugars isn't thought to have any strong links with disease.[21] [22] Another way to think of it is this: how do you think your body would fare if you predominantly lived off any of your favourite foods? Say, even, that your favourite food was broccoli and this made up the bulk of your diet. Would there be any negative effects? The short answer is probably yes. Eating a diet of mostly broccoli is likely to mean you miss out on many essential nutrients (and calories) that you need to keep your body functioning at its best.

Myth busting: does sugar feed cancer?

In the 1920s German physiologist Otto Warburg showed that cancer cells can rewire their metabolism, allowing them to ferment sugar (without oxygen) as a way of meeting their high energy demands (essentially bypassing the normal energy production seen in healthy cells, which uses oxygen).[23] More recently, this has led to claims that sugar feeds cancer, fuelling its progression and hindering people's chances of survival. But does it? And could cutting sugar out of our diet (e.g. following a high-fat, ketogenic diet) help to slow or even cure cancer?[24]

'Cancer' is often referred to as one disease, but there are many different types of cancer, which can differ vastly in the way they grow, spread and respond to treatment. Even cancers that share the same name can be vastly different. So it's complicated. When it comes to sugar, diet and cancer, things are also not straightforward.

Currently, there is no evidence that eating carbs puts you at a higher risk of getting cancer. But what about low-carb diets as a cancer treatment? Although there are animal studies that suggest reducing carbohydrates in the diet *might* be beneficial for some cancers, human evidence is extremely limited, and scientists are still (rightly) sceptical. This is partly due to the low quality of evidence we have in people (meaning results may just be down to chance) and partly due to the extreme nature of the diets used in treatment, which are exceptionally difficult to stick to. And although there have been some positive outcomes, results so far have also been mixed, with some trials finding no effects and others showing that ketones may actually drive certain cancers. So things on the science front are far from clear cut.[25] [26] [27]

▶

It 'might' be that, in the future, we learn that a diet lower in carbohydrates could work alongside chemotherapy for some types of cancer. However, as of yet, we just don't know and the stakes are high. Undertaking a diet like this with a cancer diagnosis (or not) is not without risks and has the potential to make things much worse. Cancer specialist and registered dietitian Andrea Davis agrees, 'If we cut out sugar from our diet completely it would be very restrictive and would likely lead to unwanted weight loss, which is not recommended in cancer patients, especially those undergoing cancer treatments. This is because it can worsen side-effects of chemotherapy, cause muscle loss tiredness and at worst, can result in treatments being stopped early or not working as well as they could do.'

Bottom line: You don't need to cut out sugar to avoid or treat cancer.

Important note: **Never** ditch important, proven medical therapies in favour of diet as a cure-all and always ignore the advice of anyone trying to lead you down that path. Always speak to your medical doctor and dietitian before making any dietary changes.

Is sugar addictive?

Craving sweets? Binging on carbs? Is chocolate your stress crutch? Your lifelong sweet tooth may lead some people to suggest that you have an addiction to the sweet stuff. Food addiction is a longstanding (but controversial) topic, based around the idea that food can be addictive, like drugs. Within this framework, it's been suggested that sugar could have the same addictive potential as substances like caffeine or nicotine, causing repeated overconsumption and poor health.[28] To be clear, this is not a fringe theory, it's one that regularly makes the mainstream media, with Channel 4's latest (unqualified) diet guru comparing the addictive nature of sugar to cocaine live on national TV, in September 2018.[29] [30] Anecdotally this idea is reinforced, with people left, right and centre sharing the hold that sweet foods have over them and their frustration at the lack of control they feel around these foods. What's the deal?

To understand if there is a case for sugar addiction, we first have to define exactly what 'addictive' means. Addiction is a complex phenomenon that includes social and behavioural patterns and compulsions (like pathological gambling). However, in substance abuse, the term is generally used to describe a neurobiological mechanism, meaning the addiction is the *direct* result of a chemical acting on the brain. Regularly consuming the chemical will therefore result in the hallmarks of dependency; loss of control around a substance (in this case sugar), repeated use/overuse despite negative consequences, tolerance, withdrawal and cravings. In other words, if sugar is indeed addictive, the pathological drive to eat sugar is a biological one and not something that can be overcome by willpower.

Let's see what the science has to say.

The case for sugar addiction

For sugar to be addictive, the first thing it needs to be is biologically rewarding. And it is. Both human and rat studies have shown that sugar lights up the reward centres of the brain, stimulating the release of the chemical transmitters dopamine and opioids, which make us feel pleasure.[31] Other addictive substances, such as nicotine, alcohol, cocaine and cannabis, also activate the same reward system in the brain, as do other behaviours that are linked to our survival, such as other foods and sex.[32] [33] This release of dopamine means our bodies are rewarded for sugar intake, i.e. we see sugar as a 'good' behaviour, which leads us to seek it out more.

Over repeated exposures, the sugar addiction theory goes, our dopamine receptors 'downregulate', i.e. we develop a tolerance to sugar and need more to get the same 'hit' of pleasure, leading to overconsumption and feelings of withdrawal when we stop eating it. One study that is often used to support this theory linked higher body weights with fewer dopamine receptors – suggesting that maybe higher weights were due to pathological overeating and addictive behaviours ... but this doesn't give us the full picture.[34]

The proposed sugar addiction cycle

Eat sugar $\longrightarrow$ Crave more sugar $\longrightarrow$ Develop sugar tolerance (need more sugar to get same feelings of pleasure) $\longrightarrow$ Quitting sugar leads to withdrawal.

The case against sugar addiction

Most of the evidence for sugar addiction comes from animal studies, which provide the evidence for the mechanism suggested above. However, results from human studies show a far from clear picture. In fact, although the study mentioned above was a landmark in its time, other studies since have failed to consistently find an association between weight and dopamine receptors, meaning that weight isn't a good predictor of food/sugar addiction. Further to this, a key part of the sugar addiction theory is that people with the condition will have a strong anticipatory response (their brain tells them they want the food and the food will be really good), followed by a blunted reward response (not as much pleasure as you'd expect), which leads to overeating in search of the high. Studies examining this theory are rare, but those that have been carried out also haven't shown that this is always the case. Overall, the general consensus on this topic is that despite its popularity as a theory, the current evidence to support it is quite weak, with many unanswered questions. This is unsurprising really, when you think about it. Although the idea that sugar lights up reward centres in our brain sounds like we might be onto something sinister, it's worth remembering that food is supposed to be rewarding and habit-forming – that's what keeps us going back for more and keeps us alive! Furthermore, unpicking the relationship between the chemical and emotional responses to sugar is bound to take a long time, especially as the symptoms of sugar addiction mimic those of eating disorders like binge-eating, which could explain people's responses and feelings around high-sugar foods.[35]

Myth busting: refined versus unrefined sugar

Since hating on sugar became a thing, refined sugar-free is something we find ourselves talking about a lot. There are now a ton of sugary alternatives on the market, labelled as 'refined sugar-free', advertising themselves as a 'healthy' alternative to the white stuff. We're talking about date syrup, honey, coconut sugar, agave syrup, etc. Those who tout their health benefits claim they are more natural, more nutritious and will have less of an impact on blood sugar. Let's have a look at some

▶

of these sweeteners to see if they do indeed offer a healthier alternative:

Coconut sugar is made from the sap of the coconut palm tree and looks like finely granulated brown sugar. Like table sugar, coconut sugar is a free sugar and both products contain the same number of calories. Some bloggers claim its healthy on the basis that it has undergone slightly less processing than refined table sugar and therefore contains some micronutrients such as vitamins and minerals. But, to be blunt, if you're getting a significant amount of these nutrients from coconut sugar, you're eating too much sugar!

Honey is a sweet, viscous food produced by bees. It's a sugar-based sweetener that contains a mixture of both the sugars glucose and fructose. There is some interest in honey-containing additional compounds, such as antioxidants and antibacterial agents, especially manuka honey. However, although anecdotally some people swear by its medicinal effects, there is not much evidence currently to support the clear benefits.[36] Plus, it's worth noting that honey can vary considerably in its composition, meaning the manuka honey found on the supermarket shelves is highly unlikely to be the same as the honey used in research.

Yacon syrup is quite a unique sweetener, made from concentrating the juice from the roots of the yacon plant, which is traditionally grown in the Andes. It has a caramel-like taste and a consistency like black treacle. What makes it interesting is that 50 per cent of this product is made up of prebiotic fibres, inulin and fructo-oligosaccharides, the rest being glucose and fructose.[37] Prebiotics resist digestion in the gut and they are thought to help friendly bacteria thrive and contribute to healthy stools.[38]

▶

Agave syrup is made by the liquid called agave nectar from the agave plant. This is then processed into a concentrated, sugary syrup. This modern production method means the resulting syrup sold in our stores (even the 'raw' version) bears little resemblance to the agave nectar which is touted to have health benefits. This sweet syrup is very high in a single sugar called fructose. Proponents of agave syrup claim it's low GI and therefore healthier than sugar. This is partly true, because agave syrup is high in fructose (and lower in glucose) and so has less of an effect on blood glucose levels. But GI is only one of the many things to look at when assessing the healthfulness of a sweetener. Eating a large amount of fructose, a sugar that is mainly processed in the liver, has been linked to metabolic disturbances such as contributing to insulin resistance.[39] Agave syrup contains more calories than sugar, but being sweeter means you might use less. However, overall its promotion as a natural, healthier alternative to sugar is unfounded.

Bottom line: Refined sugar-free is not a synonym for 'healthy'. All these sweeteners are fine to use if you enjoy them, but as free sugars we shouldn't be adding them to our diet for their claimed health benefits. Any benefit from additional nutrients they contain (such as in coconut sugar) is outweighed by all the sugar you'd have to eat to get a meaningful amount.

Artificial sweeteners

If you like sweet things, you might have tried sugar substitutes, or sweeteners. These sweet-tasting, low-calorie (or calorie-free) compounds, which are often referred to as artificial sweeteners (think aspartame, saccharin, sucralose and stevia), have been around for almost a century and are found in all sorts of products from low-sugar 'diet' foods and drinks, to sweets, chewing gum, fizzy drinks and toothpaste.[40] They confer to the products that contain them exactly what you'd think – sweetness (usually without the calories that come with regular sugar). They are, in fact, much, much sweeter than table sugar, with the level of sweetness in commonly used sweeteners ranging from 200–300 times sweeter than table sugar (stevia), to 37,000 times sweeter (Advantame).[41] Over the years, concerns have been raised about the safety of sweeteners, with claims of the negative effects ranging from derangement of hunger signals and weight gain, to increased risk of diseases like cancer and diabetes. Let's take a look and see if any of these claims stack up.

How do we know that sweeteners are safe?

The most well-known sweetener is probably the one with the worst reputation. Aspartame is often found in diet drinks, chewing gum and some foods marketed as health foods or diet products, such as protein bars or low-calorie ice cream. In the press, aspartame has been linked to cancer, seizures, lupus and memory problems (to name just a few).[42] So what gives? Why is such a controversial sweetener approved as safe? And how do we know it is?![43]

Despite the scare stories, there is caution applied by scientists when assessing the effects of artificial sweeteners on human health. Each sweetener undergoes scrutiny, and in Europe they are only licensed if they manage to pass safety approval tests set by the European Food Safety Authority. They do this in a very specific way. First, scientists look at long-term animal studies to calculate the highest daily dose at which no negative effects are observed when consuming a particular sweetener. This figure is called the No Observable Adverse Effects Level (NOAEL). This is followed by a second step where scientists take one-hundredth of the NOAEL to arrive at a comparatively tiny lifetime dose that they could be confident would be safe for people to consume every day. This is called the Acceptable Daily Intake (ADI), which is the maximum amount considered completely safe for us to eat every day over the course of a lifetime. If we put the above steps into practice, the NOAEL for Aspartame is 4 grams per kilo of body weight per day (and the ADI level is 40 milligrams per kilo of body weight per day). This is the equivalent to 2,400 milligrams for a 60 kilograms adult, *per day*. Since an average can of Diet Coke contains 180 milligrams of aspartame, an adult would need to drink a whopping 13 cans (nearly 4.5 litres) every day over a lifetime before reaching the ADI.[44] Remember still, even if someone did manage to drink this much Diet Coke, every day for the rest of their life, the dose of aspartame consumed would still be one-hundredth of the NOAEL, which is the highest experimental concentration of sweetener without any known adverse health effects. Despite these sweeteners having the potential to be toxic, they appear in foods and drinks in such small concentrations that we have no real chance of getting anywhere near the toxicity threshold. It's the dose that makes the poison: just because something has the potential to be toxic, doesn't mean it is. Drinking large-enough amounts of water would be toxic. We don't worry nearly so much about consuming too much vitamin A from liver, selenium from Brazil nuts or mercury from tuna fish, despite the gap between the amount we consume on average and level of toxicity being far smaller.

Do sweeteners mess with our appetite?

While artificial sweeteners are generally considered safe from a toxicity point of view (at the level consumed by the general population), do they make us hungrier? It's been suggested that the intense sweetness of sugar substitutes could act on the part of the brain involved in our appetite and food intake, messing up our bodies natural signalling and making us feel hungrier than we otherwise would. The theory is that when the brain detects sweetness without the usual calories it comes with, it recalibrates and increases our appetite, causing us to eat more to make up for the deficit. However, studies investigating this tell us this probably isn't the case.[45] A meta-analysis of short-term, randomised, controlled trials confirmed artificial sweeteners don't seem to affect people's total calorie intake; people given foods or drinks sweetened with artificial sweeteners were found to eat fewer calories compared to those eating foods/drinks containing sugar, not more.[46] So if you're choosing foods with artificial sweeteners, this isn't something you really need to worry about.

Can artificial sweeteners upset the balance of our gut bacteria?

The balance of bacteria in the gut is thought to play a major role in keeping us healthy, with 'good' bacteria lowering the risk of gut infections, producing beneficial nutrients and even supporting the immune system.[47] One of the main reasons why artificial sweeteners were thought to be harmless was that they pass through the digestive system (and out of the end) unchanged, so it was long assumed that they didn't have any effects on the body whatsoever. More recently, animal studies have challenged this assumption, suggesting that they may in fact have some effect on our body, via our gut bacteria. One study, for example, found that when mice were fed an artificial sweetener called saccharin, the species and numbers of bacteria were altered, including a reduction in beneficial varieties.[48] Another study in mice found this alteration in the microbiome led to glucose intolerance (pre-diabetes).[49] In people, some observational studies indicate that those who eat artificial sweeteners have a different gut bacteria profile to those who don't[50], but these studies can't say for sure if cause and effect is at work here and it's too early to jump to conclusions! Conducting high-quality human studies in this area of nutrition is tricky and, currently, we don't have any good human trials that can give an indication of cause and effect. It may well be that some populations of bacteria thrive from using artificial sweeteners as food, whilst others dwindle from its toxic effects.[51] The full extent to which artificial sweeteners affect our gut health isn't fully understood, so what we need now is more research.

Do artificial sweeteners interfere with our blood sugars?

There are concerns that eating sweeteners such as saccharin, aspartame and sucralose could change the way the body handles sugar, leading to poor blood sugar control and an increased risk of diabetes. The premise is that the intense sweetness from these sweeteners activates 'sweet-taste' areas in the gut (which respond to the sugar we eat or drink), increasing the absorption of any sugar eaten into the blood. The jury is currently out on this one. A recent systematic review concluded that the way the body handles sugar in response to eating sweeteners is unclear, due to studies producing contradictory results.[52] Some showed blood glucose increased in response to eating sweeteners, some showed blood glucose decreased and others showed sweeteners had no effect. What's really needed here is further research with comparable, well-designed studies looking into the effect of different sweeteners on blood sugars and, importantly, determining who (if anyone) might be at risk.

Some sweeteners (mainly the sugar alcohols such as xylitol) have a health claim approved to say that replacing sugar with these sweeteners reduces the rise in blood sugar after a meal. However, there is not enough evidence to say that replacing sugar with sweeteners will manage blood glucose levels better overall.[53]

Do artificial sweeteners cause weight gain?

Another worry is that artificial sweeteners (e.g. in diet drinks) can lead to weight gain. Recent studies have determined an element of reverse causality is at play here; this is where one element causes another, but not in the way suggested. Therefore, in the case of artificial sweeteners, it's not the consumption of artificial sweeteners that cause the weight gain observed. It has therefore been proposed that those with a higher body weight are more likely to be on a diet and therefore more likely to be drinking sugar-free soda, rather than artificially sweetened drinks leading to increased body fat.

The overall body of evidence currently suggests artificial sweeteners are safe, do not cause cancer and, if you already include them in your diet in moderate quantities, there is no concrete evidence you should stop. But nothing is 100 per cent certain in science and there are grey areas – such as their effect on the gut – which justify further probing. Keep in mind that swapping sugar with artificial sweeteners doesn't automatically mean something is a health food. They might help you reduce the amount of calories you consume and allow you to eat sweet things whilst protecting your teeth (especially if you usually eat a lot of sugary foods), however, adding stevia to a cookie doesn't make it broccoli!

Is consuming artificial sweeteners risky? The answer is, based on what we currently know and the amounts that people are consuming in their day-to-day lives, most probably not. As it stands, although they may not be completely biologically inert, the risks have been blown out of proportion, with many of the wild claims being extrapolated from the animal and test-tube research and applied to people – which isn't good science!

Does sugar cause acne?

Managing acne through diet can be a confusing journey, replete with old wives' tales and contradictory advice. Does chocolate cause spots, or is it ok? What about dairy? Or sugar?

The *exact* cause of acne is unknown, but dermatologists believe factors such as hormones, weight, genetics, inflammation and emotional stress play a role. The British Association of Dermatologists describe the oil-producing glands of people with acne as being particularly sensitive to normal blood levels of key hormones, causing glands to produce excess oil.[54] Skin cells lining the pores may also not shed properly, causing follicles to block. This combined oily and blocked-pore environment causes the acne bacteria (which live on everyone's skin) to multiply.

▶

The role of diet in acne development has only recently re-emerged as a topic amongst scientific literature, albeit it is still viewed controversially. A review reported that milk, chocolate, pizza, the Western diet, glycemic load and low-fat milk have all been foods of interest.[55]

A recent systematic review found that the majority of studies looking into diet and nutrition are of poor quality, with almost 90 per cent of the literature being level D evidence (opinion pieces or case studies)[56]. This is perhaps because, compared to drug studies, nutrition studies are difficult to conduct, being tricky to blind, as well as expensive. But registered nutritionists, dietitians and dermatologists should be open-minded and aware that they may be able to make a small impact on someone's life by improving their skin with food in the context of improving their overall diet quality (when used alongside proven medical therapies). Hopefully we will see more collaboration between both professions in years to come.

Nutrition recommendations

If you feel that your diet is linked to having flare ups in your acne it might be worth starting a food/symptom diary to look for patterns between foods and breakouts. If you do this, please discuss it with your GP or Registered Dietitian to ensure you aren't implememting unnecessary restrictions.

Top tips for acne management from Dr Anjali Mahto, consultant dermatologist

- Choose skincare products that contain the following ingredients: salicylic acid, glycolic acid, niacinamide, zinc, tea tree oil and retinol. These can help reduce inflammation and reduce blockages with the pores.

- Don't pick or squeeze your spots as this can result in scarring or infection.
- Make sure you cleanse your skin twice a day, both morning and evening.
- Consider using a targeted spot treatment containing salicylic acid overnight to help dry out your spots and reduce inflammation.
- If your spots are getting worse despite using appropriate skincare for several weeks, starting to cause scarring or affecting your mental health, it is time to seek help from a medical professional such as your GP or dermatologist.

6

Protein

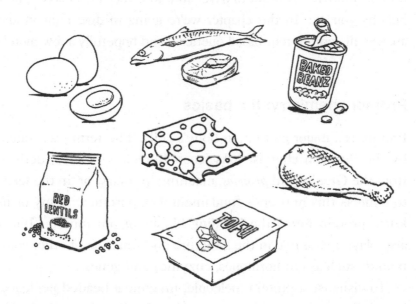

Unlike fats and carbs, everyone seems to agree that protein is important. And they're right. Proteins are made up of smaller molecules called amino acids, which are, quite literally, the essential building blocks of life. We need them for everything – from facilitating the chemical reactions that keep our bodies functioning, to building our muscles and organs, to forming the structure of our DNA. The focus on the importance of protein has changed quite noticeably in recent years; it's no longer seen as a nutrient that's only relevant to bodybuilders and athletes, moving into the realm of positively mainstream. People are starting to think more

about it, asking questions like, am I eating enough protein to promote optimum health? How much do I really need? Does it matter
when I eat it? Is it better to get my protein from plant sources or
from animals? Should I be using protein powders and are they
healthy? Is too much bad for your kidneys? The list goes on!

On average we eat more than enough protein to avoid deficiency,
but the actual amount that you need is quite individual. It depends
on several factors, including your age, activity levels, the amount of
muscle you have (or want to have) and, in a very broad sense, how
healthy you are. In this chapter we're going to dive right in and
answer all your protein-based queries – and hopefully a few more!

Protein chemistry: the basics

Protein is a major part of our body's cells. The term was coined
by the Swedish chemist Jöns Jacob Berzelius in 1938, derived
from the Greek word *proteios*, meaning 'primary' or 'in the lead',
to express this nutrient's fundamental importance. Many of us
know protein forms the building blocks of our muscles but it
also plays a vital role in the structure and function of other compounds such as our hormones, enzymes and genes.

To visualise a protein molecule, imagine a beaded necklace;
just as the necklace is made up of beads, the protein molecule
is made up of smaller molecules called amino acids. There are
20 different amino acids in nature and, just as a beaded necklace
can be made up of different types of beads (plastic, glass, metal),
a protein molecule is made up of hundreds, or even thousands
of the 20 different amino acids, laid out in a unique sequence.
This unique sequence and the fact that the protein chain can be
folded into different shapes is what gives each of the millions of
proteins its own individual properties.

Essential and non-essential amino acids

In the late 1930s, an American scientist called William Rose conducted a famous set of studies on rats, introducing the idea that some amino acids are more important than others. In his experiments he fed rapidly growing young rats a controlled diet, containing fat, carbohydrates, vitamins, minerals and a source of protein that contained all 20 of the amino acids. He then methodically removed single amino acids from the diet, one at a time, and observed what happened. The removal of some amino acids didn't make a difference to the rat's development or health, but the removal of others dramatically halted the rat's development and eventually resulted in weight loss and death. Rose then did a similar experiment on humans and discovered which amino acids are required in our diet. He found that more than half of the 20 amino acids in proteins are what's known as *non-essential*, meaning the human body can make them itself. Although we can find these amino acids in food, it's not essential that we do so for our health. However, there are nine amino acids that adult humans can't make and must be eaten in the diet (histidine, isoleucine, leucine, lysine, methionine, phenylalanine, threonine, tryptophan and valine, to be specific!). Interestingly, some amino acids are considered to be essential under certain conditions, such as childhood, illness or stress (aka conditionally essential amino acids).

How much protein do we need?

The body is constantly making protein (by stringing together amino acids) or breaking it down, as needed. Unlike carbs and fats, we don't have a place to store protein in the body (muscle doesn't count as a storage facility), and since our bodies need to use protein every day we have to replace these losses by eating. If our diet didn't provide adequate protein to replace these losses, we would quite literally digest ourselves, starting first with our muscles and, in severe cases, our organs such as heart muscle.

How much protein do I need?

It's currently estimated that a healthy adult requires about 0.8 grams of protein per kilogram of your body weight each day. Luckily most of us in the Western world tend to meet our protein requirements easily. This is because food is relatively accessible and most people eat protein in such large amounts that they receive all the amino acids they need. Even those who are very active don't necessarily need much more – as long as their diet provides enough food to meet their increased energy needs, their protein requirements should be met. An average man or woman could easily meet their protein needs by eating porridge made with milk for breakfast, a chicken sandwich for lunch and a veggie bean stew with rice in the evening. A chicken breast has relatively large amounts of protein but there are plenty of good sources of plant-based protein (such as beans and legumes), and even though grains and vegetables contain much less, they can significantly contribute to the daily protein intake if eaten throughout the day. People who are recovering from an illness/surgery, are elderly or very active might have higher protein needs than average.

When should I eat my protein?

Bodybuilders have been using nutrient timing as part of structured eating plans to maximise muscle gains for decades, and it's thought of by many people in the sports industry as an essential component of an athlete's training, specifically to promote performance and muscle building. But is it necessary? The short answer is no. Although protein is best distributed throughout the day, rather than eaten in one go (because the body can only process and utilise a certain amount of protein for muscle protein synthesis at one time), this is something we all do quite naturally anyway and isn't something that you need to worry about. Additionally, although some people (particularly those in the fitness world) obsess about pre and post workout rituals, including protein timing, most of the research in this area has been done in elite athletes and isn't applicable to the rest of us mere mortals. Even for athletes trying to build muscle, research generally shows that the most important thing is getting enough protein, not when it is eaten.[1] So whether you're a gym lover or not, simply eating protein regularly throughout the day is what counts.

Protein concerns

Although protein hasn't been vilified in the same way as carbohydrate or fat, there are some questions about protein that pop up quite regularly – so let's take a look.

Is meat bad for me?

Headlines often vilify red meat and processed meat, but are they really that bad?

Red meat is the muscle meat from mammals such as cows, pigs, horses and sheep.[2] It's red when raw and tends to go darker when cooked (as opposed to meats like chicken, which are white). But should we eat it?

One of the main concerns about eating meat is that it causes cancer. This is an unsurprising fear, given that it's a narrative that has received a lot of attention in the media, especially since it featured in the popular (but wildly misleading) documentary *What The Health*. It's not a completely unfounded claim, but it's a prime example of the nuance required when talking about nutrition and health.

The World Cancer Research Fund has concluded that red meat has a 'probable' (as opposed to 'convincing') link with cancer. However, although this may be true, we need to exercise some caution when interpreting this as a public health message. Red meat is nutritious (and delicious) and can absolutely form a healthy part of a balanced diet (if you want it to). For example, although red meat has been linked with cancer in observational studies, some dietary patterns containing small amounts of red meat, such as the Mediterranean-style diet, have been linked with health effects.[3]

One difficulty we have when examining the evidence for meat and health is that if you eat a lot of meat, the *type* of meat you eat may be important, but many studies don't separate red meats from processed meats. One huge observational study that did manage to do this, however, was the EPIC study. Researchers looked at the data and aimed to determine what, if any, links there were between red meat, processed meat (and poultry) with risk of early death.[4] Nearly half a million healthy men and women provided information about their diet and were observed by scientists, who tracked them for up to 17 years. The researchers found that while processed meat was linked to an increased risk of death, red meat was not. Interestingly, in the EPIC study, the lowest risk of death was found in the group who ate a moderate amount of red meat, not the group who ate the lowest.

Processed meat is meat that's had 'stuff' done to it to extend its shelf-life or change its taste, such as salting, smoking or curing. These meats include bacon, salami, chorizo, sausages, dried meat (e.g. beef jerky), cured meat and canned meat (like corned beef). Processed meat has also been linked observationally with a range of chronic diseases such as heart disease, diabetes and, most notably, bowel cancer. There is consistent, convincing evidence that shows that bowel cancer is more common in people who eat the most red and processed meats. Most of these studies are the type that can't prove processed meat causes disease but can show a relationship exists. However, there are studies showing that consumption of red and processed meat increases the production of compounds that can cause cancer (the effect is worse when the diet is low in fibre and if large amounts of red and processed meat are consumed).[5] The World Cancer Research Fund's latest report has also confirmed there is 'convincing' evidence that a link exists (we discuss the meaning of this link in more detail in the plant-based chapter). It's worth bearing in mind with observational data like this that other factors come into play. People who eat lots of processed meat may have other lifestyle characteristics that mean they are at higher risk. This idea has been highlighted in research which suggests higher processed-meat-eaters are more likely to smoke and eat fewer fruits and vegetables compared to those eating smaller amounts.[6] Scientists do try to correct for these confounding factors in their studies, but these methods are not foolproof and it's possible this could partly explain why such an association exists.

So according to the science, eating meat, particularly processed meat 'might' increase your risk of bowel cancer. However, your overall risk will be influenced by your whole dietary pattern and lifestyle. So a bacon sarnie at the weekend is probably not going to make a huge difference.[7]

Is too much protein bad for my kidneys?

The kidneys are incredible organs which filter the blood and helps remove waste and fluid from the body as urine. Some scientists have concerns that a high-protein diet (like the Atkins diet) requires the kidneys to filter a strenuous amount of protein. The worry is that over the long term, this strain might cause more serious damage and result in chronic kidney disease. Kidney specialist, dietitian and researcher Dr Helen McLaughlin told us, 'Overall, studies looking at the effect of high-protein diets on kidney function in the short term have not found any detrimental effects when kidneys are working normally and are undamaged.[8] However, the effect of a high-protein diet over months to years is still not known.'[9]

The type of protein is also worth mentioning. Dr McLaughlin highlighted, 'Eating diets high in animal-protein foods may not be helpful for people who already have damaged kidneys.' It's potentially the type of protein that could be important for protecting the kidneys in healthy individuals, too. One study looking at the effect of different protein foods in healthy individuals found replacing red and processed meat in the diet with alternative sources of protein (such as nuts, legumes and low-fat dairy) was associated with a decreased risk of developing kidney disease.[10] More studies are also needed to confirm these findings – a recent review found there is a real absence of evidence[11] – but it seems a sensible idea to include more plant-based protein in the diet as the evidence currently stands.

Protein in practice

So that's the basics. But how do we put this all together in real life?

Protein quality

A 'high-quality protein' contains all the essential amino acids in relatively the same amounts and proportions that human beings require; it may or may not contain all the non-essential amino acids. Proteins that are low in an essential amino acid cannot, by themselves, support protein synthesis. Generally, foods derived from animals (meat, fish, poultry, cheese, eggs, yoghurt and milk) provide high-quality proteins. Proteins from plants (vegetables, nuts, seeds, grains and legumes) have more diverse amino acid patterns and tend to be limiting in one or more essential amino acids, meaning you must eat a wider variety of them to cover all your bases, so to speak. Plant proteins can also vary quite widely on the number of amino acids they contain; for example, some plant proteins are also notoriously 'low quality' or don't have a wide variety (such as corn protein). A few others are high quality and contain many more (such as soy protein). Although speaking of protein sources in this way makes it seem as if plant-based proteins are 'inferior' to animal ones, it's important to point out that it's just a term for quantifying the variety of essential amino acids available in a single source and that it's perfectly possible to get all the protein you need from a plant-based diet if that's how you choose to eat.

Complementary proteins

Since plant-based proteins generally don't contain all the essential amino acids, it's recommended for vegetarians and vegans to combine two or more different plant protein foods with complementary amino acid profiles to create complementary proteins, thus ensuring the body is provided with all the essential amino acids in the diet. While it's long been believed necessary to do this at each meal (for example, combining brown rice with legumes), this is not really necessary in practice. As long as sources of protein are mixed up throughout the day and the diet provides enough energy, most healthy vegetarians or vegans will avoid protein deficiency by enjoying a variety of beans, whole grains, nuts seeds and legumes.

AMINO ACID GRID

	ISOLEUCINE	LYSIN	METHIONINE	TRYPTOPHAN
LEGUMES	▨	▨		
GRAINS			▨	▨
TOGETHER	▨	▨	▨	▨

For example, in general, legumes are rich in the amino acids isoleucine and lysine but fall short in methionine and tryptophan. Grains have the opposite strengths and weaknesses, making them a perfect match for legumes.

Protein food sources

Animal sources

- Beef.
- Chicken.
- Pork.

- Lamb.
- Fish.
- Eggs.
- Dairy: milk, yoghurt, cheese.

Processed meat (any meat that has been smoked, salted, fermented, cured or undergone any other process to alter its flavour or shelf life.)

- Ham.
- Salami.
- Bacon.
- Some sausages (frankfurters and chorizo).

Plant-based sources

- Soya and soya products, e.g. tofu, soya mince and soya dairy alternatives.
- Beans, lentils and chickpeas.
- Seeds.
- Nuts and nut butters, e.g. peanuts or almond nut butter.
- Whole grains.

Talking point: protein powders

Nichola Ludlam-Raine, specialist registered dietitian

If you're meeting your daily protein requirements through your diet (diet here referring to the foods and drinks that you already consume), you do not need to take a protein supplement. If you're not meeting your protein requirements (which you probably are),* protein supplements, often sold as ready-made drinks, powders and bars, can be a convenient, low-calorie and low-volume way of helping you meet your protein needs; after all, how easy is it to carry a chicken breast with you to the gym, in comparison to a ready-to-drink protein shake?

Whey protein (often sold as a ready-to-mix powder) is one of the most popular protein supplements on the market and is derived from the water-soluble part of milk. All protein breaks down into amino acids in the body, with specific amino acids such as leucine acting to encourage muscle growth. There are 20 different types of amino acids, nine of which are essential, meaning we have to get them from our diet as our body cannot make them. Whey protein is considered a 'complete protein' as it contains all nine essential amino acids; so if you do require a protein supplement to meet your protein needs, it might be a useful addition to the diet. Whey protein is absorbed relatively quickly, so as well as helping with muscle growth alongside exercise, it can help to preserve lean muscle tissue when losing weight or during the natural ageing process.[12]

Current protein intake recommendations for non-athletes, endurance athletes and resistance-training athletes are 0.8 g/kg per day, 1.2 to 1.4 g/kg per day and 1.6 to 1.8 g/kg per day, respectively.[13]

* Average protein intakes in the UK exceed the requirements.[14]

7

Micronutrients and Supplements

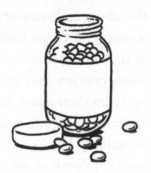

Micronutrients are important vitamins and minerals that we require in tiny doses. They play a key role in our body's cells and organs. They are also crowned 'essential nutrients' in our diet, which means our body can't magically create them, so we need to get them from food or we risk developing a nutrient deficiency. But how can we ensure we're getting enough? We tend to have a 'more the merrier' attitude to taking vitamins because nutrition in a pill seems so alluring – the ultimate nod to letting 'food be thy medicine'. Before we look into who might benefit from supplements, let's go way back, centuries ago, to find out how this interest in vitamins and minerals all came about.

The discovery of vitamins

Let's go back a couple of hundred years, to a time where people suspected food contained something special, something vitally important for life, but couldn't quite put their finger on it. Scurvy is a good example of how this thinking progressed. This disease, causing sore limbs, weakness and bleeding gums, resulted from a lack of vitamin C and was estimated to have affected two million sailors.[1] A clever chap called James Lind conducted a trial of six different treatments for 12 sailors with scurvy and found that only oranges and lemons were effective in treating the disease. By the end of the eighteenth century, British naval ships were made to carry a supply of citrus fruits. People knew this treatment worked, but they didn't know why and it wasn't until the turn of the twentieth century that the reason for this was discovered. They were given their name by a biochemist called Casimir Funk in 1912; *vita* meaning life and *aimine* being a word relating to the protein building blocks amino acids (which they were thought to contain).[2] A flurry of activity then followed in the labs, as scientists raced to synthesise vitamins themselves. Ten Nobel Prizes were awarded for research into vitamins between 1929 and 1943, and by the 1950s, vitamins were being created in labs and added to foods to enrich or fortify them.

Prior to this, diseases such as scurvy and rickets were considered by some to be infectious or as a result of a toxin – not a lack of nutrition! Also, the main food philosophy of Funk's era was that only four components of nutrition were necessary for good health: protein, carbohydrates, fats and minerals. But, thanks to the painstaking contributions from different scientists to solve each vitamin puzzle, we live in a world today where we have the ability to prevent and treat micronutrient-related disease. When supplements were brought in from the 1930s onwards, they were advertised as an answer to deficiency diseases and a way to keep illness at bay.

We now have a fully blown supplement industry on our hands. This is without a doubt booming, being set to be worth £158 billion globally by 2022.[3] And while hoping to benefit from a healthy glow, it's not just vitamin C we can pop, it's also minerals, enzymes, fibre, herbs, bee pollen, spirulina and green tea. All these can be taken as pills, but also as powders, sprays, shots and in reformulated food. Hands up who has used supplements as a safety net for lifestyle slip-ups in the past? It's perhaps the miraculous effects seen following reintroducing a deficient nutrient that has led many of us to assume consuming them in supplement form (often in vast quantities and combinations) can cure a range of ailments.

Micronutrient chemistry: how are they measured?

We only need micronutrients in teeny amounts. Instead of grams, they're measured in smaller units: milligrams (mg) or micrograms (µg).

1g = 1000 mg

1 mg = 1000 µg

Vitamins: why do we need them?

The body needs 13 different vitamins to support specific functions in the body that promote growth, repair and the maintenance of life. Although vitamins do not directly provide energy when broken down, they assist the body's enzymes to yield energy from the digestion of carbs, protein and fat.

They can be divided into two main groups: fat-soluble and water-soluble. The difference between these groups determines how each vitamin acts in the body.

Water-soluble vitamins C and B complex

These vitamins are found in a wide variety of foods, albeit in relatively small amounts. Our body does not have a storage facility for these vitamins, which means you pee out any excess (the orange, energy multi-vitamin Berocca will make your wee bright yellow due to the presence of B2, aka Riboflavin).

Fat-soluble vitamins A, D, E, K (mnemonic: All Day Eating Kake)

These vitamins are found in a smaller variety of foods, most of them fatty and some of them in pretty high concentrations. Liver for example contains a large amount of vitamin A. The body can store vitamins A, D, E (and B12) in amounts to last for months or even years, which means you may not need to get these vitamins from your diet daily.

Minerals matter too

Minerals come from non-living stuff, like rocks and earth. If you're familiar with the Periodic Table from your chemistry lessons, you'll know what we mean when we say minerals are elements. Think iron, magnesium or calcium. Although plants contain minerals, they only do so because they have absorbed them from the earth! The amounts required range from grams per day (like sodium or potassium), to a few micrograms per day in the case of selenium. Those needed in smaller amounts are sometimes known as trace elements. And luckily, since minerals are present in most living things, it's difficult to get deficient in them when following a normal balanced diet. But deficiencies do arise, particularly in areas where the diet is restricted to foods growing in mineral-depleted soil, or if someone has a gut disease (such as a coeliac) where they might have problems absorbing certain nutrients. Minerals are also pretty robust. Unlike vitamins, which can be destroyed by heat or air, minerals are more resilient and will only be lost via cooking if they leach into cooking water like the water-soluble vitamins.

Nutrient losses

As soon as fruits and vegetables are picked, the nutrient-loss clock starts to tick. The same goes for all fresh foods on their journey from farm to fork. Although cooking can improve the availability and absorption of nutrients in foods, overcooking or ineffective storage can increase nutrient losses in your fodder. Here are our top tips to keep your food as nutritious as possible.

- Keep (most) fruit and vegetables in the fridge.
- Store cut fruit and veg in airtight wrappers or containers.
- If you need to boil your veggies, add them once the water has already reached boiling point, and cook for a short amount of time. Or, even better, steam your veg in a small amount of water or microwave them (contrary to popular belief, micro-waving doesn't 'kill' the nutrients in food).
- Don't be afraid to buy frozen – the freezing process maintains the nutritional value of the vegetables!

A deeper dive into some key micronutrients

Vitamin D

Why do we need it? Helps to regulate the amount of calcium and phosphate in our body, which is vital for strong bones and muscle.

Food sources: Oily fish, dairy, egg yolks, red meat, liver, fortified margarine and breakfast cereals.

Tip: The best source of vitamin D is sunlight (between the months of April and September) or supplements. Most people in the UK should consider taking a 10mg supplement daily during the winter months.

Vitamin C

Why do we need it? Helps to protect our body's cells and keep them healthy. Deficiency may cause thickening of the skin, poor wound healing and a severe lack of it can lead to scurvy.

Food sources: Oranges, lemons, kiwi, blackcurrants, mangoes, papaya, guava, peppers, broccoli, Brussels sprouts, sweet potatoes, liver and kidney.

Tip: It's easy to get enough vitamin C via a healthy balanced dict. You can reach your daily requirements via eating just half a red pepper.

Iron

Why do we need it? Enables red blood cells to carry oxygen around our bodies. A poor iron intake can lead to iron deficiency anaemia, which can make you feel tired and breathless.

Food sources: Liver, meat, poultry, fish, eggs, beans, nuts, dried fruit, whole grains, fortified breakfast cereals, yeast extract, green leafy veg.

Tip: The iron found in animal-based foods compared to plant-based is more easily absorbed into our bodies. Having food or drink high in vitamin C at mealtimes alongside iron-rich plant foods increases the amount of iron that is absorbed. Polyphenols such as tannins found in tea and coffee may reduce the amount of iron you absorb, so if iron is a nutrient of concern, try to avoid drinking these one hour before and one hour after your meals.

Folic acid (folate)

Why do we need it? Folic acid is important for the production of healthy red blood cells and reduces the risk of neural tube defects in babies while they're developing in the womb.

Food sources: Folic acid found in food is called folate. This is found in most fruit and vegetables (especially green leafy vegetables), beans, peas, fortified breakfast cereals, whole grains, nuts, dairy products, eggs and meat.

Tip: It is recommended to take a 400-milligram supplement if planning a pregnancy, up until the twelfth week of gestation. Women who aren't pregnant or planning for a baby should be able to get all the folate they need by eating a varied and balanced diet.

Iodine

Why do we need it? Iodine is involved in the production of thyroid hormones, which help to keep our body's cells and metabolism (chemical reactions in the body) healthy. An iodine imbalance can lead to an overactive or underactive thyroid.

Food sources: Fish, shellfish, seaweed, dairy products and iodised salt. Iodine can also be found in plant foods such as cereals and grains, but the levels vary depending on the amount of iodine in the soil where the plants are grown.

Interesting fact: In many countries, iodine is added to table salt (called iodised salt) to increase its intake. This is not done in the UK, where the nation's iodine intake rose following the addition of iodine to cattle feed in the 1930s, which in turn increased the iodine concentration of milk. This was done to improve the health of the cattle, not humans. Without a formal iodine-fortification policy in the UK, iodine intake is dependent on an individual's food choice, leaving certain groups of people vulnerable to iodine deficiency.

Tip: It can be difficult to get enough iodine if you don't eat fish and dairy, particularly in pregnancy. Some women may benefit from a supplement, ideally starting three months prior to getting pregnant. These should only be taken with medical supervision. Kelp or seaweed supplements can provide excess iodine, so these should be avoided.

B12

Why do we need it? Involved in releasing energy from food, making red blood cells, keeping our nervous system healthy and using folic acid. Not getting enough may cause harm to the nervous system, which can lead to limb weakness, numbness or tingling, and in some cases problems with memory and brain function.

Food sources: Meat, fish, eggs, dairy, yeast products (such as Marmite and nutritional yeast), fortified breakfast cereals.

Tip: If you include meat, fish or dairy food in your diet, you should be able to get enough B12. Vegans may struggle as B12 is not found naturally in foods such as whole grains, fruits and vegetables, or in spirulina (contrary to popular belief).

Calcium

Why do we need it? Most of the calcium in our body is used to make strong bones and teeth. It's also important for muscle contraction and blood clotting. Low intakes in childhood can stunt growth, increase the risk of brittle bones, rickets in childhood or osteoporosis in later life.

Food sources: Dairy, fortified dairy alternatives, green leafy vegetables, beans, lentils, chickpeas, tofu, nuts, bread, tinned fish (with bones).

Tip: If you don't eat dairy, be aware that organic dairy alternatives (such as organic nut milks) are not allowed to fortify their products with additional vitamins and minerals.

To supplement or not to supplement

The market for dietary supplements is booming with millions of people in the UK supplementing their diet with the hope of improving their health or staving off disease.[4] In fact, if you have a health concern, you can probably find a dietary supplement designed to help, a neatly packaged solution to a complex problem. But do they work?

Do I need supplements to be healthy?

The busy, fast paced lives that many of us lead can make supplements an appealing quick fix, especially if we are feeling tired and run down. But although vitamins and minerals support normal good health in our bodies, they don't provide the same health benefits as whole foods and they're not a silver bullet. Whole foods deliver a range of micronutrients, working together in a complex synergy, taking part in thousands of chemical activities throughout the body. This is why a key component of good health is eating a variety of these foods, something supplements just can't compete with.

Many of us take a multivitamin 'just in case' – a sort of insurance policy against what we might or might not eat, so that all bases are covered if our diet is sub-par. But is this worthwhile? A large review looking at 27 vitamin trials concluded that people who took vitamins were not necessarily healthier. In the 400,000 people included in the review, the vitamin-pill consumers did not live longer or have fewer cases of chronic diseases like cancer or heart disease compared to people who did not take them.[5] Studies have also found taking supplements could be harmful. Vitamin E supplementation, for example, has been linked to an increased risk of lung cancer in smokers. A 2012 systematic review looking at over 87 randomised controlled trials concluded that evidence does not support the use of antioxidant supplements, either in the general population or in those with various diseases.[6] They specifically mentioned there was a slight increased risk of death from taking beta-carotene and possibly vitamin A and E, but not vitamin C or selenium.

Overall, from a science perspective, supplementing with vitamins and minerals hasn't been linked with any meaningful benefits. Unless you have a deficiency or struggle to get certain nutrients from your diet due to restriction (e.g. veganism) or poor health, then getting your vitamins and minerals from a balanced diet is considered best.

Some to consider, some to avoid

Supplements to take or avoid	
Consider taking daily	**Avoid**
Vitamin D Due to poor sunlight in the UK winter months (and lack of good vitamin D food sources), everyone should consider a daily 10µg supplement in winter months	Multivitamins and/or antioxidants For the majority there is no benefit in taking these. They are not only likely to be ineffective but may put your health at risk
For specific needs Folic acid For women trying to conceive and advised for pregnant women to reduce their risk of neural tube defects in their baby	Fat-burning or slimming pills Especially containing DNP (Dinitrophenol) or DMMA (Dimethylamylamine), which can be extremely dangerous to human health and can even lead to death
B12 For vegans, as this vitamin is found in eggs and dairy foods (although fortified foods could be eaten instead of supplementing)	Fish liver oil Should not be taken by pregnant women as vitamin A can be harmful to babies in large amounts
Algae-derived DHA For those who don't eat fish (e.g. vegans and some vegetarians)	Vitamin E Should not be taken by those with heart disease as it can increase the risk of further heart attacks
Probiotics If you're prone to traveller's diarrhoea or have been on antibiotics	

Myth busting: IV nutrition therapy

This has been touted by many celebs as a quick way to make you feel better, support your immune system, hydrate you, prevent disease, cure jet lag, brighten your skin, improve your mood and all sorts of other health benefits. And it sounds kind of sensible, right? Vitamins are good for you, we need them, they are 'natural', so they are probably harmless and having more should be better. Also, they are given in some clinics by

▶

doctors and nurses, so they seem backed by medicine, so they must be legit?

But that's sadly not the case. Our first issue with this practice is that IV drips carry an unnecessary risk of infection. If your gut is fully functioning there is no reason to take this risk, as oral vita-min supplements are known to be effective for correcting vitamin and mineral deficiencies. Only people with a severe deficiency, or a condition that means they are unable to absorb the vitamins in their gut are likely to require IV replacement (under medical supervision).

Secondly, the places giving these therapies often aren't checking your blood to see if you need them. Many such clin-ics screen and recommend a vitamin cocktail based only on a lifestyle questionnaire. This means that you don't know if you are deficient in any of the vitamins and minerals they are advising you take. As they are likely to be water-soluble vitamins, this means your kidneys will just filter out the excess you don't need and you will pee them out. It's just a recipe for very expensive wee.

Additionally, as many clinics don't test your levels beforehand, in some cases the doses they are giving you could be quite risky – especially as many clinics advise you to have a 'course' of mega doses, which could leave you with very high levels of some minerals, outside of the normal range. Finally, this practice is not regulated and practitioners don't need to be licensed.

Our take-home message? Scientists have consistently found that supplements are no replacement for a healthy, balanced diet, and getting nutrients from whole foods is the ideal option. However, if you are deficient or at risk of missing a specific nutri-ent, taking a supplement could be beneficial.

8

Balanced Eating

Silver bullet (noun): a simple and seemingly
magical solution to a complicated problem.

Balance. It's a term that is bandied about as the solution to all fads and quick-fixes. Health professionals use it like it has a hard-and-fast definition, weight-loss companies dress their rule-laden plans up as a balanced lifestyle rather than a diet and fitness regime and health bloggers claim to embody it with their love of exercise and avo-heavy brunches and occasional 'guilty treats'. But balance isn't a number of calories or a macro count or a dietary pattern. It can't be found between the complicated statistics of a science journal, nor in the musings of a social media post, where it's offered up as a bite-sized set of rules: 'have one square of chocolate, just don't eat a family sized bar'. It's not 'being good' by depriving yourself of what you enjoy for a lesser, low-fat, low-sugar option at the supermarket, and it's definitely not exercising as a punishment for eating.

So what the hell is it?

The concept of balance is, to be honest, both brilliant and incredibly frustrating. It embraces all aspects of food, from the need for nutrients to the need for comfort and the joy of food-centred celebrations. It allows you to take care of your body and to eat foods you love and enjoy. It acknowledges that sometimes you will eat until you are uncomfortably full and other times you will skip breakfast. It's the concept of exercising for the sheer joy of the way it makes you feel and skipping training days to sit around in your PJs and eat cake, if that's what feels right. Most importantly, balance looks different on everyone, which is why it can't be packaged and sold as a meal plan or fed to you in bite-sized chunks through Instagram memes.

Many people find this frustrating as they just want to know what to do. The ambiguity of balance, coupled with strong differences in opinion about what constitutes an optimal diet and which foods promote good health, can for many only contribute to the confusion that surrounds food. For a moment, consider this. With all the rules and 'wearables' and tracking and counting and eating on the run, somewhere along the line we've lost the art of eating. The faith in our own ability to choose foods that nourish our bodies and at times, our souls, because eating isn't just a perfunctory task, a chore we participate in to ensure we keep on living. Food *is* life; we need it to provide the nutrients to keep us healthy, but on so many more levels than physical existence.

The foods we eat can influence our health. That is undebatable. However, what is often not explained is that diet makes up just one tiny portion of 'healthy'. Health in the current age is billed as something you work for – that you can buy in the right supermarkets or have the right gym membership. It's got its own 'look', promoted by the fitness industry: thin, white, able-bodied, six-pack, labelled gym gear or 'goals'. However, health isn't, despite what we are sold, something that sits neatly inside our own individual control. Working as a dietitian 10 years ago you had to emphasise diet to get people to take notice that it might be important. Now we have the opposite problem – people are *so* focused on their diet they forget that there are many other factors that contribute to our health. Many things impact our health, including our genetics, our environment, stress, financial and food security and housing, to name but a few. Although we strive to keep our bodies in top condition and stave off poor health and disease, the reality is, lifestyle-based prevention is not perfect.

The World Health Organization (WHO) defines the social determinants of health, or the ones that are dictated by our environment, as 'the conditions in which people are born, grow, live, work and age'. Many people reading this book will have vast privilege in this area; they will have a roof over their heads, food on the table, a job and a steady income. If you're in all those categories, you're already doing well in the health risks department. In fact, one of the biggest risks to people's health is poverty and yet we place a large emphasis on food and diets as single causes and determinants of disease.

Our obsession with eating perfectly puts us at risk of developing unhealthy, polarising attitudes to the food we eat and getting too caught up in the trivial. We live in different environments, have different genetics and what works for one person might not work for another. One great example of this can be seen in the blue zones. These regions (namely Sardinia, Italy, Okinawa, Japan and Loma Linda, California) are pockets around the world where people live remarkably long and healthy lives. Although the diets of people in these regions share many qualities, e.g. based on fresh, whole foods, they're also not the same. Some are higher in fat, others higher in carbs and they all have their own cultural quirks – from seaweed to olive oil or sauerkraut – that make them unique. This simple observation teaches us one of the most important lessons we can learn about nutrition: there's not one perfect diet that promotes optimum health, but rather some repeating overlapping features that point to the basics of a healthy balanced diet.

Scientists have noticed there are some basic, consistent lifestyle patterns that these communities share. They seem to foster a healthy relationship towards food; they don't generally cut out food groups or demonise individual nutrients. They don't worry about the proportion of protein, fat or carbs they're eating, and they don't take a concoction of nutritional supplements every day. They eat seasonally and in accordance with their culture. Perhaps most tellingly, their lifestyle is also more than good nutrition: they don't smoke (generally) and enjoy regular, low-intensity activity. They engage with their society and are surrounded by others living in the same way and have a sense of faith and purpose. These basic principles make up the cornerstone of their healthy lifestyle. The logical conclusion we can draw from this is that healthy people can maintain their health on a variety of diets, despite our desire to search for the perfect way to eat. We may naturally choose some foods over others due to food availability, personal preferences and needs, but this should be celebrated and embraced.

What is the Mediterranean Diet?

A healthy community you've probably heard of before are those living in the Mediterranean. There's often lots of talk about the Mediterranean diet in the media, but what does eating in this way really look like? This style of eating is based on the traditional foods eaten by people in countries like Greece and Italy in around the 1960s. In the years following World War II,

▶

American scientists were surprised to find that the relatively poor population in Crete were extraordinarily healthy compared to Westernised Americans. Notably, these people were poor but had much lower rates of diseases such as heart disease. This discovery motivated researchers to dig a little deeper into the diet and lifestyles of these people, which is where they stumbled upon what's now outlined as the Mediterranean-style diet. Since then there have been randomised controlled trials and large epidemiological studies that reported associations with lower rates of heart disease.

Importantly, there is no one strict definition for this diet. The Mediterranean is full of distinct populations and they didn't traditionally all eat the same thing. The diet is also not necessarily what you see if you visit Mediterranean countries today (although we do love eating pizza!). That said, most definitions include lashings of extra virgin (cold-pressed) olive oil, vegetables including leafy green vegetables, fruits, cereals, nuts and pulses/legumes, moderate intakes of fish and other meat, dairy products, eggs and red wine. It's fresh and simple.

The take home here is that when it comes to food, we need to look at the bigger picture. Healthy diets can look very different – the wider circumstances in which we live play a huge role in determining our health status and finally, food is so much more than its constituent nutrients, it's an important part of the social and cultural fabric of our communities.

Context matters. No diet is perfect. What does balance look like for you?

A food-based guide to eating well

Add in:

- Fruits and vegetables: choose a wide variety, in lots of different colours, including beans and legumes.
- Seafood (including a portion of oily fish per week).

Switch to:

- Plant-based protein sources (e.g. legumes, beans, nuts, tofu and tempeh).
- Foods that contain mostly unsaturated fats (e.g. olive oil, olives, nuts, seeds, oily fish).
- Whole grains: choose whole-grain options when you eat bread, pasta, breakfast cereals and grains such as rice.
- Unsweetened dairy products.

Choose less often:

- Sugary drinks, sweets, pastries and other products containing lots of free sugars.
- Processed meat.
- Fried foods.

Graphic for a healthy diet

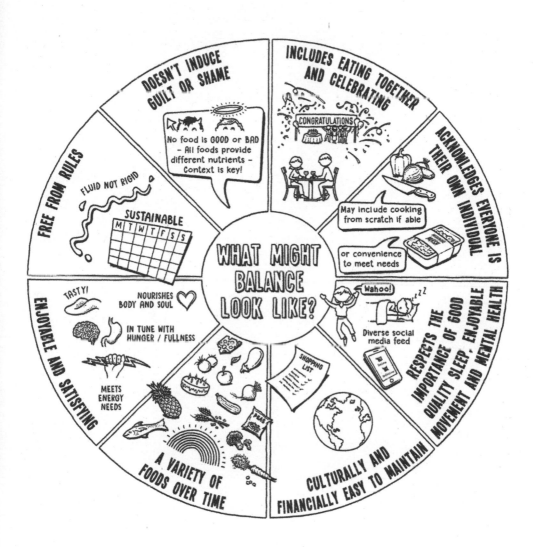

Plant-based Eating

Nutrition advice may seem to be constantly changing (depending on who you're listening to and which diet they are advocating for), but if there is one thing that everyone – even experts with conflicting favourite dietary patterns – can agree on, it's that eating plants is good for your health. The popularity of plant-based eating has risen dramatically over the last few years, with more and more people considering both the health and environmental impacts of the food they choose to put on their plates. However, the term itself can be a little confusing and its increasingly widespread use has thrown up a few big questions, so let's dig a little deeper and look at what plant-based eating actually means and how eating more plants is good for both your health and that of the planet.

What is plant-based eating?

Despite most people believing that only vegans can truly call themselves plant-based, when people say they follow a plant-based diet it may mean they choose to follow one of a number of different dietary patterns. The fact is the term has no hard and fast definition, so you may be a vegan, vegetarian or flexitarian plant-based eater, but whichever describes you, if you're plant-based, your diet places plants at the front and centre, making them the star of the show. Plant-based eating is a diet that is based *primarily* on plants (as opposed to only on plants), although it's commonly used interchangeably with reference to veganism. So, for the purpose of this chapter and context, what we mean as dietitians when we say plant-based is this; if your diet is derived mainly from plants, or in practical terms is based around vegetables, whole grains, nuts, seeds, legumes and fruits, with either small amounts of animal products or none at all, you could describe yourself as a plant-based eater.

What's so special about plants?

Plants are pretty amazing. They are a source of vitamins and minerals, as well as plant compounds such as flavonoids and polyphenols. They also contain plant proteins, dietary fibre and healthy fats, all of which are thought to contribute towards keeping our bodies healthy. As we have discussed in other chapters, the complexity of 'health' and all the different factors that influence it, means that it can be difficult to determine a cause and effect relationship between food and disease. (That's why you should always be wary of headlines like [insert food here], causes cancer.) However, what we do know is that people who have diets that contain lots of plant foods tend to have lower risks of certain diseases than people who eat a Western diet that is high in refined carbs and low in plant foods. If you think this sounds quite vague, you'd be right! But remember, science (especially nutrition science) isn't about 'proving' stuff, it's about trying to limit doubt and reduce our chances of making false connections.

There are other studies that back up the theory that eating more plants reduces your risk of diseases like heart disease and cancer. These are called 'mechanistic studies', or put more simply, studies carried out in test tubes and on animals that test a theory by exploring how an effect might come about.

Here are some of the ways in which scientists think plants could work to improve our health:

Reducing inflammation

Inflammation (in the most basic sense) is a defence mechanism that involves your body's immune system. It occurs when your body recognises something as harmful (maybe a toxin, or a disease-causing bug, or damaged cells) and it responds to this threat by trying to remove it and heal itself. In fact, your body wouldn't be able to heal itself without inflammation. (Think about cutting your finger, the red, swollen, throbbing feeling is your body directing blood flow to the area to neutralise the threat.) However, inflammation can also be a bad thing. An inability to remove a harm or change a situation that is putting stress on your body can result in long-term inflammation, which occurs silently within your body and can last months and even years. This is sometimes called chronic inflammation and it is thought to be a major factor in the development and outcome of many diseases, including heart disease, diabetes and some cancers.

Eating plants can help to reduce chronic inflammation through the anti-inflammatory effects of some of the compounds they contain, such as vitamins and polyphenols (beneficial plant compounds). The way they exert these effects is quite complicated (and to be honest, unless you like reading long lists of words you can't pronounce, the mechanisms are a bit dull), but in

simple terms, they suppress the compounds that activate inflammatory pathways in the body.

However, it's worth noting that although plants provide compounds that are thought to have these effects, this is something
that occurs over a long period of time. This is often misrepre-
sented in the communication of this concept, especially in relation
to health foods. So in practical terms, what this means is sporadi-
cally dosing up on 'superfoods' touted for their high antioxidant
content or drinking a turmeric latte to counter a boozy night out,
kind of misses the point. To maximise the anti-inflammatory
effects of plants, you need to eat them often and think about the
balance of your diet over the long term and not as a quick fix.

Oxidative stress

Some of the compounds in plants are thought to reduce oxida-
tive stress,[1] which is caused by an imbalance of compounds
called free radicals in the body. These compounds are missing
an electron (a particle that gives atoms a negative charge), so
they are very unstable. Think of them as an unsupervised tod-
dler at a party, charging about, nicking other people's toys or
forcing the toys they don't want onto other people. That kind
of chaos. These unruly compounds are either formed in our
body during normal metabolic processes or introduced via our
lifestyle and environment, through things like smoking. Again,
much like toddlers, the free radicals you produce in your body
actually aren't all bad. They are used in small amounts in some
processes in our body, for example, some immune responses.
However, if there is an imbalance of free radicals, where there
are too many for our body to control and disable, they can cause
damage to our body's cells. Antioxidants such as vitamin C
from plant foods can be helpful for ridding us of any excess free

radicals, protecting our bodies from damage. However, when it comes to antioxidants, 'more' isn't necessarily better. In fact, we make a lot of antioxidants inside our bodies to ensure we have a defence against free radicals, but although eating lots of plant foods can provide us with antioxidants alongside other helpful plant compounds, supplementing with 'extra' antioxidants hasn't been shown to be helpful for reducing our risk of disease and, paradoxically, in some cases it's even been shown to be harmful. For example, high doses of the antioxidant beta-carotene has been linked to an increased risk of lung cancer in smokers. Bottom line? Eating antioxidant-rich plant foods is good for your health. Supplementing with them, not so much.

Improving gut health

As discussed in more detail in our 'gut health' chapter on pages 149–177, feeding the bacteria in our gut with a variety of dietary fibres from plant foods helps to maintain a healthy, diverse range of bacteria in your gut. Eating fewer plants, which is common in our 'Western-style' diets, is associated with a less diverse gut flora and, subsequently, poorer gut health and higher risk of disease. Having lots of fibre also means you're more likely to have regular, healthy bowel movements. More plants = better poop!

Detoxification enzymes

Some of the compounds in plants, such as phytochemicals, might be able to alter the process of converting and eliminating toxins from our body.[2] Generally speaking, this may mean that certain foods, such as cruciferous vegetables, might help to support our body's in-built detox systems, optimising their function. However, this is a new area of research and more studies are needed before we can put this information into practical advice. Additionally, given the complex interactions between the individual chemical components of plant foods, the best way to support your body's detoxification systems is to eat a wide variety of vegetables.

Plant synergy

One of the things that's interesting about plants and health is that although many people have tried to isolate 'healthy' compounds from plants, package them and sell them, the benefits seem to be very much attributable to the 'whole food' rather than isolated nutrients.[3] Foods such as nuts, whole grains, fruit and vegetables are consistently associated with lower disease risk, but when the components from foods that we think are beneficial are studied on their own, we don't see the same benefits. This is likely because the ways in which plants confer a health benefit are due to complex, synergistic contributions from interactions within the food structure. In more simple terms this means that although there is some cool stuff in there, these foods are more than the sum of their parts – when you put them all together, they are much more powerful. In science we can see this as studies investigating isolated compounds, such as antioxidants, show fewer benefits than the whole foods. This means it's not possible to mimic the effects of a diet rich in fruits and vegetables in special superfood powders or supplements and the best way to experience the health effects of fruits and vegetables is to eat them whole.

How many plants should I be eating each day?

Something we get asked a lot is how many plant foods we should be eating for optimal health, but the truth is, it's an impossible question to answer. The actual amount of anything that you need to eat is very personal; it depends on your choice of dietary pattern, activity levels, health status – we could go on. Even advice on fruits and vegetables varies from country to country (mostly because this advice is based on what is 'health promoting and achievable' for the general population, rather than for optimal health). However, what we do know is that, in general, people who eat more fruits and vegetables tend to be at a lower risk of disease than people who don't.

Let's put this into context.

There have been lots of different studies showing that eating more fruits and vegetables is associated with a lower risk of diseases like heart disease and cancer. Recently, a group of scientists from Imperial College London pulled all these studies together and conducted a hugely powerful meta-analysis that combined the data from lots of different studies (a total of around two million people!) to see if they could more definitively see the relationship between fruits and vegetables and health. What they found was the more fruits and vegetables people ate, the lower their risk of some diseases, right up to a whopping 10 portions a day (that's where all the headlines came from!). The stats from the study showed that people who ate 10 portions (or 800g) of fruits and vegetables a day had a 28 per cent lower risk of heart disease, a 33 per cent lower risk of stroke, a 13 per cent reduced risk of cancer and a 31 per cent reduction in dying prematurely.

Powerful stuff.

But does this mean we should all be eating 10 portions of fruits and vegetables a day? Maybe. Remember that this is based on observational data, and even though there are signs that the link could be causative (the effects were strong, even after other factors that could influence results had been corrected for, consistent between studies, and we have a plausible mechanisms to explain them), the information we got from this study wasn't only that

'10 might be best'. One of the most interesting things about this and other studies in this area is that the biggest benefits are seen at the lower intakes of fruits and vegetables. What this means is someone who eats one portion of fruit and veg per day and increases that to five will see a bigger reduction in disease risk than someone who goes from five to eight. Just try to do your best.

We will also see in the gut health chapter that the diversity of your plant-food intake is just as important for gut bugs and gut health. Eat your fruit, veg and other plants, but you don't have to be hitting double figures to make a difference. Mix it up – every little helps.

Five-a-day – What counts?

Contrary to popular belief, five portions of fruit and veg isn't the optimal amount we should be aiming for per day, it's actually what scientists believe is the minimum amount needed to be eaten daily to experience significant health benefits. Other countries have different figures: Japan aims for seven, Greece aims for nine! Just aim for more – include any fruit or veg you can to get to your five-a-day (or 'more-a-day'!)

A portion is:

- 80 grams of whole fruit or veg (frozen and canned count, too) OR
- 30 grams dried fruit and veg.

Some portions can only count once:

- 150 millilitres fruit or vegetable juice or smoothie (see the sugar chapter for why this is).

▶

- 80 grams beans and pulses (these are a great source of fibre but contain fewer nutrients compared to whole fruit and veg).

Common beans and pulses:

- Lontils.
- Adzuki beans.
- Chickpeas.
- Red kidney beans.
- Butter beans.
- Black-eyed beans.
- Soya beans.
- Cannellini beans.
- Peas.

Eleven ways to plantify your plate

1) **Fold in your greens:** Not everyone fancies a serving of steamed kale on their plate. Instead, you can think about shredding, folding, wilting. Shred your greens (cabbage, Swiss chard, spring greens, spinach or kale) and fold them into your stews, pasta, grains, risotto – anything that's warming in a pot. When the greens hit the warmth, they wilt, sneakily pushing up the plant power in your dish.

2) **Think beyond beef:** You don't have to go veggie to eat more plants, but you can think about reducing some of the meat in your meals and substituting it for plant-based protein. Swap half of the meat in a stew for beans or legumes and add some tinned tomato for extra flavour.

3) **Salad is more than iceberg:** A salad does not have to be just a standard lettuce chopped up with a quartered tomato. Think about rainbow colour and crunch. Try different salad leaves, add grated carrot, toast some seeds, chuck in some roasted veggies or sprinkle with fresh herbs. The possibilities are endless, but the key is to mix it up with variety. Even think of this as a bolt-on, a side dish to really help maximise your fruit and veg intake.

4) **Big batches:** Set some time each week to do some batch cooking. Chop up a handful of different veggies and roast until slightly charred and caramelised. Store in a Tupperware in the fridge for easy access when adding to a breakfast omelette, a sandwich at lunch or to bulk up an evening meal.

5) **Mix it up:** No one plant food is star of the show. Diversity is key, so try to move away from having the same fruit and veg on rotation. How about adding a new fruit or vegetable to your repertoire each week? Stick a seasonal fruit and veg calendar on your fridge and get creative.

6) **Harness the hummus:** Hummus and any other bean-style dips are a delicious way to get more plants on your plate, whether it's as a dipping vehicle, soup topping or a creamy filling to your sandwich. They're also incredibly easy (and cheap) to make if you have a hand blender or food processor.

7) **Colour half your plate:** It can be easy to forget about plants when we're so used to meat being the star of the show. A useful prompt to ensure your veg intake is at its best is to fill half your plate with two different types of veg.

8) **Frozen is your friend:** Before it reaches your supermarket shelves, fresh produce needs to be picked, packaged and transported. This takes time, and during these hours (or days) nutrients can be lost. Frozen fruit and veg is frozen within hours of picking, sealing in its nutrients. A recent study testing the vitamin content of eight different types

of fresh and frozen fruits and vegetables found the frozen foods contained comparable or even higher amounts of vitamins compared to the fresh stuff.[4]

9) **Meat-free Monday:** This is a fantastic campaign launched to inspire people to ditch the meat on Mondays. It's a simple way to increase your plant-food intake without feeling overwhelmed at each meal. Just focus on one day and take it from there.

10) **Swap your spuds:** We love the humble potato, but it doesn't count towards your five-a-day. How about occasionally swapping these out for other veg that do count? Sweet potatoes, parsnips and beetroot are delicious roasted or mashed. You could even try half and half in some mash.

11) **Go bananas at pudding:** Fruit for pudding does not need to be boring. Baked bananas, stewed fruit or poached pears can be jazzed up with creamy, crumbly or nutty toppings.

Myth busting: are organic crops more nutritious?

James Wong, botanist

The idea that organic crops contain higher levels of vitamins and minerals is an extremely common claim in the media. Dozens of studies have found that crops grown according to organic principles *do* contain higher levels of key nutrients and these findings are often enthusiastically reported in the press. But there is one small flaw in this narrative: an equally large number of trials, it appears, have found the exact opposite to be the case. In fact, even within the exact same crop, studies often report that while

▶

some nutrients appear to be slightly higher, the levels of other vitamins and minerals are lower. This creates a body of data that is so heterogeneous and filled with contradictions that it can be extremely tricky to draw meaningful conclusions from it.

One of the reasons for this is that making like-for-like comparisons between organic and non-organic crops is notoriously difficult. In addition to having been grown according to different agricultural practices, they are also likely to be totally different genetic varieties, grown in different countries, with completely different soils, weather and even transport and storage techniques – all of which can dramatically affect the outcome and skew the results. To find an accurate answer to this question scientists have to sift through all the available data out there from dozens of studies, collating it together in one place to see if they can find meaningful patterns in the evidence. A mammoth number-crunching challenge. Now, this has been done three times by different independent universities and in each of these cases the researchers were not able to find any reliable evidence for consistently higher (or lower) levels of vitamins and minerals in organic crops. In fact, these levels are so naturally variable it is impossible to say whether the growing method has any impact at all.

What we *do* know, however, is that organic crops tend to be more expensive than their conventional equivalents, sometimes substantially more. The bottom line is, if you want to choose organic and can afford to do so, you are extremely unlikely to be missing out in the nutritional stakes. But if you are doing so because you believe paying a little extra means you will be rewarded with a proportional increase in nutrient content, well, this is not a claim that is supported when you look at the best evidence we have to date.

Veganism

Once considered to be the realm of hippies and far-left liberals, veganism is now more popular than ever. It's quite difficult to say how many people are actually vegan in the UK, but a survey carried out by the Vegan Society in 2016 estimated that the number had risen to over half a million, which is around a 350 per cent increase from 2006 – a trend that has been reflected in surveys from other parts of world, including Canada, the US and Australia. There are now vegan bodybuilders, pro-athletes and celebrities, and with the rise of the conscious consumer, the interest in the lifestyle seems here to stay. However, like any movement with a cultural and ethical agenda, vegan lobbying gives rise to a large amount of conspiracy and misinformation (both for and against the diet), especially when it comes to nutrition and health. If you're interested in objectively exploring a vegan diet, let's look at the facts.

Vegan diets contain absolutely no animal products, excluding foods like honey as well as the obvious ones – meat, fish and dairy products. Anecdotally, many people rave about the healthfulness of their vegan diet, and it's true that it can be useful for increasing your intake of protective plant compounds and beneficial nutrients, mostly because vegan diets are usually high in plant-based foods such as vegetables, fruits, grains, nuts and seeds. In fact, vegan and vegetarian diets have been linked with lots of health benefits, especially when compared to the average Western diet, which is low in plants and high in processed meat. This includes a reduced risk of certain diseases, including heart disease, type 2 diabetes and some cancers. In fact, one study reported that vegetarians (which included vegans) have as much as a 32 per cent reduction in their risk of heart disease compared to non-vegetarians.

Wait. Surely this means they are 'healthier', right?

Not so fast. Results from these studies have been mixed and are far from conclusive. Remember that observational studies, by their nature, can't tell us WHY vegans have a lower risk of some diseases, or what causes this link. So it could be their diet, or it could be something else.

Vegans and vegetarians are likely to be quite health-focused people, and in general the ones who have been studied are more healthy living beings than the general population.[5] While it might be the elimination of meat and animal products that gives them these shiny stats, it could also be because they are from a wealthier section of society who are less likely to smoke and more likely to participate in healthy behaviours. People from higher socio-economic groups often have more access to healthy food and safe places to exercise, greater amounts of time (and facilities) to cook, more family and social support and exposure to lower levels of stress – all of which impact our health. Additionally, most of the research looking at vegans and vegetarians versus meat eaters has failed to show that vegans live longer. In fact, the 2015 Oxford EPIC study, which followed more than 60,000 people in the UK, found no statistical difference in death rates between vegans, vegetarians and meat-eaters. This might be (again) because volunteers for the studies were all relatively healthy people (meat-eaters and vegans alike), so there weren't enough deaths overall for the researchers to be able to see a benefit from vegan diets. However, the bottom line is that, as it stands, we don't really know if vegans live longer, or if they do, if it's because of their diet.

What's our view on a vegan diet?

We've had a lot of stick for saying this, particularly from vegan activists, but – 'deep breath' – here goes: all these things mean is that a well-planned vegan diet can be a really healthy diet, but it's definitely not the only healthy diet.

Glad that's out of the way.

Overall, vegans tend to eat more plants, which means that going vegan can help people increase the amount of healthy fibre, nutrient and plant compounds they eat, providing health benefits.

However, it's important to remember that you don't need to be a strict vegan to eat less meat and more plants. It's not the LABEL that makes your diet healthy, it's your dietary habits. Think about this for a second; just going vegan or vegetarian doesn't mean your diet will automatically become healthier, it's way more complicated than that. In fact, a US study in 2017 pooled together the data from three very large observational studies (>200,000 people) to see if they could find any link between diet and heart disease.[6] On their initial analysis, they were surprised to see that there wasn't much difference in risk between plant-based diets and meat-containing diets and risk of heart disease. However, when they looked at the data more closely and separated out those eating an 'unhealthy' vegetarian diet, which included lots of refined grains and sweets, from those eating a 'healthy' vegetarian dietary pattern, which was high in whole grains, fruits, vegetables and healthy fats, those eating an 'unhealthy' veggie diet had a higher risk of heart disease. Whereas, as expected, those eating a higher quality diet had a lower risk.

Healthy vegan dietary patterns certainly seem to have benefits, they have been linked with a lower risk of heart disease and cancer.[7] The BROAD study, a six-month randomised controlled trial, sorted people with one or more of the following: type 2 diabetes, heart disease, high blood pressure and high cholesterol, into either normal medical care for their condition plus a whole-food, plant-based diet or just normal care.[8] They found that those following the whole-food plant-based diet with twice-weekly support from healthcare professionals significantly improved all health markers, including cholesterol levels, blood pressure, blood glucose control (without prescribing calorie restriction or exercise).

However, the health benefits listed above are not unique to vegan diets. We've seen similar benefits from dietary patterns that feature plants heavily, like the Mediterranean[9] and Nordic[10] dietary patterns. To us, this means that although there are some good reasons to go vegan and that switching to a plant-based diet can provide some people with some serious health benefits (especially if they are following a poor-quality Western-type diet), it's not a necessity for good health. Following a vegan diet and getting everything you need can be tricky too – so there are some lists, which we will discuss.

As veganism has risen from a conscious movement to protect animals and the environment, there's unavoidably been a rise in conspiracy soundbites like 'meat causes cancer', or 'eating two eggs a day is the equivalent of smoking five cigarettes a day', both of which were parroted out in the famous *What The Health* documentary. It's important to think critically when hearing bold and scary statements like these.

Three vegan myths

1. Meat causes cancer: It's true that the IARC (International Agency for Research on Cancer) classes meat as a type 2 carcinogen (and processed meat as a type 1 carcinogen), which sounds really serious and scary but in fact isn't saying what it seems to be saying. These classifications refer to the *certainty* with which we know, from scientific studies, that meat is linked to cancer. It's about strength of evidence, not level of risk. It also doesn't tell us anything about how much meat increases our risk, or the amount associated with this increase. Although scientists believe the link is pretty certain (especially for processed meats), the *level of risk* is fairly small. Cancer is a complex disease that doesn't have one single cause and can be influenced by many different factors. It's also likely from a dietary perspective that your actual risk of cancer also depends on your diet as a whole,

▶

rather than the inclusion or exclusion of meat. This was reflected in the Oxford EPIC study of cancer rates in vegetarians and non-vegetarians (all of whom were quite healthy).[11] They found a small reduction in risk of all cancers in vegetarians, but a higher risk of colorectal cancer. The overall risk of cancer in both groups was very low, supporting the idea that there is more than one factor at play, and your modifiable risk of cancer is as much about what you include as what you exclude in your diet (as well as other lifestyle factors, obviously). Vegans/veggies still get cancer. (See Chapter 6, Protein, for some practical food recommendations.)

2. Eating eggs is as harmful as smoking: Eggs have had a bit of a bad rap over the years, mostly because of the high cholesterol content of their yolks. Due to the link between high LDL cholesterol levels and heart disease, many people assumed that eating fewer eggs would keep their blood cholesterol levels low, reducing their risk of developing heart disease. However, we now know that dietary cholesterol has very little impact on our blood cholesterol levels. More recently, fear about eggs was renewed when the *What The Health* documentary claimed that eating a single egg could decrease your lifespan as much as five cigarettes. This statement seems to be drawn from an observational study that found that consuming egg yolks was associated with an increased build up of fatty deposits in the arteries.[12] The researchers do not report the exact amounts that smoking affected build up in the arteries, but said that both egg consumption and smoking followed a similar, linear pattern. However, these people did not have heart disease and apart from smoking, other aspects of people's diet and lifestyle were not measured, meaning that this link could have been caused by any number

▶

of other factors. We also know from other observational studies (which showed no link between egg consumption and heart disease in healthy people) and intervention studies (which show that eggs tend to raise 'good' HDL cholesterol rather than 'bad' LDL) that eggs are a perfectly healthy choice for many of us, which is why there is currently no upper recommendation for a maximum number of eggs eaten per day in the UK.

3. Eating dairy leaches calcium from your bones: A common criticism of dairy products is that they contribute to the development of the bone disease osteoporosis. This is because some observational studies have seen that the countries with the highest intake of dairy products also have the highest incidence of osteoporosis. People who promote this myth state that this occurs due to milk being 'acidic' and causing calcium to leak out from your bones to neutralise the threat, making them weaker.[13] This theory falls down in a number of places. Firstly, it ignores the 'bone-friendly' profile of dairy foods; they are rich in calcium, protein and minerals, all of which are essential for good bone health.[14] Controlled trials also show beneficial effects, whereby eating dairy leads to improved bone health.[15] Secondly, this theory does not acknowledge the role your kidneys play in maintaining blood pH; they filter out any 'acidic' compounds and you pass them out in your urine – your bones aren't involved in this process.[16] Overall, there are many factors at play in bone health, including physical activity, diet, age and hormones. Although some observational studies have shown dairy to be potentially detrimental for bone health, their results might be clouded by other factors. In addition to this, many more observational studies have shown beneficial effects and have clinical studies to back them up.

Final note! We know that many people choose veganism for ethical reasons – and that's fantastic. If you are passionately trying to promote plant-based eating for ethical reasons, focus on the ethics, not the propaganda about health. Interestingly, most surveys have found that vegans who choose the diet for ethical reasons are more likely to stick with it than those who go vegan purely for health reasons, suggesting people are motivated more by causes that are bigger than themselves.[17] It's fair to say that (for some) switching to a plant-based diet may have some health benefits. However, remember that dietary choices are deeply personal, so if you are in a position of privilege, where food is abundant enough for you to be picky about what you eat and where it comes from, the odds of you being 'healthy' are already heavily stacked in your favour. Be kind to people and try to refrain from judging other people's dietary choices – you don't walk in their shoes.

Overall, this reinforces what we have learnt in earlier chapters of this book. There's no one road to good health and a healthy diet isn't down to the inclusion or exclusion of certain individual foods or food groups. When it comes to healthy eating, it's your dietary patterns over weeks, months and years that will make a difference, so find what works for you.

Eating well on a vegan diet

We know we've sort of slated focusing on single nutrients and a reductionist approach to health earlier in this book, but veganism is the one area of nutrition where a reductionist approach (or focus on single nutrients) can be useful. This is because there are some nutrients that are more difficult to get when you exclude animal products, and vegans need to focus a little bit on their diets and the nutrients they contain to ensure that they are getting enough of everything. Many public health bodies and dietetic associations talk about 'well-planned' vegan diets, because you need to have an awareness of where you're getting certain nutrients from and which ones you need to supplement. One example of this is calcium. As most people in the UK get most of their calcium from dairy, ensuring that you are getting enough when you've eliminated the major source in your diet is important, especially for bone health. This is demonstrated when looking at the vegans in the EPIC Oxford trial. Overall, vegans in this study had a 30 per cent higher risk of fractures compared to non-vegans. However, when the researchers looked at people who had adequate calcium intakes there was no difference in risk between people who were vegan or not. This means that if you are vegan, getting enough calcium should be a priority and careful planning can reduce your risk of fractures. Other nutrients of concern include omega-3 fats, zinc, vitamin B12, iodine, vitamin D, selenium and vitamin K.

Why some people might not do well on a vegan diet

Many people will thrive on a well-balanced vegan diet, but not all of us will. The right diet for us depends on many factors, including cost, food availability, personal preferences and health status. From an affordability and accessibility perspective, it may be that many people, (particularly in areas of the country known as 'food deserts') may lack access to the foods you require in order to ensure you are eating a balanced vegan diet that provides you with all the nutrients you need. Others may lack the time, skills and resources (such as a working kitchen) to be able to eat this way.

However, while we often recognise the social and environmental factors that limit people's dietary choices, when it comes to veganism, the science suggests that some people experience physiological limitations, too – namely our genes and our microbes. Genetic mutations mean that some people don't convert plant sources of vitamin A into the active form very well, for example.[18] Additionally, (although evidence is lacking for some of these theories) it's also been suggested that certain gut bacteria profiles may make it harder for some vegans to obtain enough vitamin K2. Although these theories are fringe, they do provide ideas for mechanisms which might explain why some people find it harder to thrive on a vegan diet.[19]

A note on eating disorders

It's unfortunate but necessary to highlight here that some people use veganism/vegetarianism (and other socially acceptable restrictive diets) to facilitate disordered behaviours or hide their eating disorder in plain sight under the guise of 'ethics' or 'health'. This is *not* to say that everyone who is vegan/veggie has an eating disorder or that veganism causes eating disorders. However, both veganism and anorexia are restrictive by nature and it can be difficult for people with an ED to separate whether they are making a choice for ethical reasons or for their eating disorder – EDs *love* restriction, it's what they feed off. Because of this, it's important to be aware of signs that your choices may be negatively impacting on your mental and physical health and unpick your motives when moving to a restrictive diet – especially if you have had an eating disorder in the past.

Know the first signs

The charity BEAT have created a useful guide to spotting the first signs of an eating disorder. If these things resonate with you

▶

and you are worried about your eating habits, then it's always best to speak to a medical professional. Although this may seem scary, BEAT have a wide range of resources on their website to help you get the right help, including a section on what to expect when you start a conversation with your doctor. They even have a leaflet you can print off and take with you to the GP to help you clearly explain your concerns.

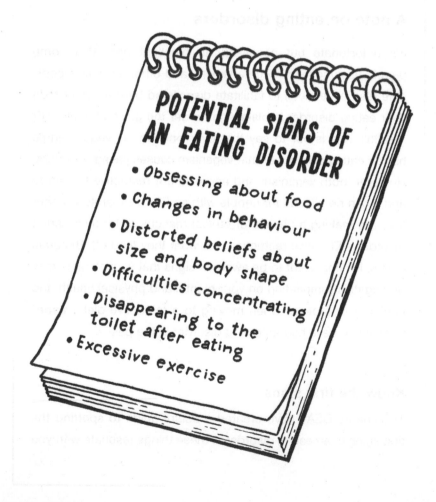

POTENTIAL SIGNS OF AN EATING DISORDER
- Obsessing about food
- Changes in behaviour
- Distorted beliefs about size and body shape
- Difficulties concentrating
- Disappearing to the toilet after eating
- Excessive exercise

Eating sustainably

Eating well for health is one area of nutrition that has had its fair share of attention. But there's a new kid on the block, creeping into people's consciousness: sustainable eating. It's not always apparent to us, in our bubble of supermarkets and online shopping, that the food we eat is intricately linked with our planet. The reasons why we choose food are complex, but they usually include its availability, cost and because we know we like the taste. This means that it's easily forgotten, when aimlessly wandering through the supermarket scouting out BOGOF offers on our favourite brands, that what we eat (quite literally) connects us with the earth we walk on and our dietary choices have an impact that stretches way beyond our own physical being.

This is changing, first and foremost because we live in a world with a rapidly expanding population. It's been estimated that we have around 218,000 new mouths to feed every single day, which is something that our current food system will struggle to keep up with in the years to come. As more people become aware of the far-reaching effects of what we choose to put on our plates and ask themselves about the environmental impact of their food, some big questions crop up – is it possible to eat a diet that matches up our health needs with those of the environment? And what is the best way to eat for protecting the planet?

'What, and how much we eat directly affects what, and how much is produced. We therefore need to consume more "sustainable diets" – diets that have lower environmental impacts and are healthier.'

Garnett et al, 2014[20]

What is a sustainable diet?

In its simplest sense, a sustainable diet is one that promotes the good health of both people and the planet. This is defined by the Food and Agriculture Organisation as nutritionally adequate, safe, healthy, culturally acceptable, economically affordable and environmentally friendly. Which means for a diet to be truly sustainable it has to tick a lot of boxes, across a range of many complex environmental and social systems. Because (generally speaking) plants tend to have a lower environmental impact than animal foods, and in observational studies vegans and vegetarians tend to experience some health benefits as a result of their dietary choices, following a vegan or vegetarian diet is often assumed to be the most sustainable way of eating, best for both health and the environment. And this assumption is made with good reason. A 2016 systematic review examined the evidence for 14 different sustainable dietary patterns and scored them based on their effects on greenhouse gas emissions, land requirements, water use and health.[21] Veganism scored very highly, coming out top for a number of sustainability markers, including reduced land use and greenhouse gases. This review also estimated that on a global scale, moving away from a Western diet towards more sustainable dietary patterns could reduce overall greenhouse gas productions from the food supply by as much as 70 per cent and water use as much as 50 per cent, which is a hugely significant amount.

However, although in general eating less meat and dairy and more plants is widely considered the best way to reduce the environmental impact of your diet, at an individual level the picture is much less clear cut. In fact, while being vegan or vegetarian certainly means you are more likely to have a sustainable diet than people who follow a Western-type dietary pattern, it's not a guarantee that your diet will be more or less sustainable than someone else with a different healthy dietary pattern (e.g. the Mediterranean diet). This is because the actual environmental impact of your diet and the food you choose can vary widely, depending on where it was grown and its production processes. Additionally, as well as factors such as food packaging, food waste, miles travelled and type of transportation, your diet has to meet your individual needs over the long term and be one that you can maintain and afford.

The environmental aspect of this variability was demonstrated in the results of a small study of 153 Italian adults, which was made up of 51 meat-eaters, 51 vegetarians and 51 vegans.[22] The researchers looked at the differences in environmental impact between the diets of these individuals, grading their diets by nutritional adequacy, greenhouse gas emissions, land and water use. What they found may surprise you. Although, as expected, overall the omnivorous diet was the least sustainable of all the diets, creating a larger environmental impact across the board, there was no difference between the environmental impact of vegans and vegetarians. Additionally, they found that there was a wide range of individual variability in what people ate, even within those with the same chosen dietary pattern. One of the most interesting observations was that even after adjusting the numbers to account for differences in energy intake, some vegans and vegetarians still had a higher environmental impact than some meat-eaters. The authors put this down to volume of food needed to meet nutritional needs, as well as food choices within the vegan diets, in particular high intakes of fats, protein and processed meat and dairy replacements.

Health and environmental factors don't always add up either. Sugar has a relatively low environmental impact compared to some foods, whereas some fruits and certain varieties of vegetables have been found in some instances to have a high environmental impact relative to some animal products. This shows that it's impossible to make the most environmentally friendly choice all of the time and we have to strike a balance between our nutrition needs, our health and the environment.[23]

Overall, if sustainability is a priority for you, the single biggest change you can make that will likely have a beneficial effect on both the health and the environment is to eat fewer animal products like meat, fish and dairy – and replace them with whole, plant foods.

Vegan and vegetarian diets are both healthy and sustainable choices that can vastly reduce the environmental impact of your diet if you can commit to this way of eating. However, there can be many reasons why people can't (or don't want to) go vegan or vegetarian and, ultimately, you don't have to strictly eliminate all animal products to make a meaningful impact. In the UK alone animal products account for over half of food-based greenhouse gas emissions. It's been estimated that the amount of greenhouse gas emissions that occur due to food production could be reduced by 40 per cent, simply by people reducing (rather than eliminating) animal products and moving towards a healthier dietary pattern, which might be much more realistic for many people.

10

Eating for a Healthy Gut

It's clear that gut health is a major trend. There's kombucha turning up in edgy (and mainstream) cafes, sauerkraut classes are replacing flower arranging and – thanks to Giulia Enders' book *Gut* – poo naturally crops up as acceptable dinner party chat. It's becoming increasingly clear to both scientists and the public that taking care of our gut may be one of the single most important things we can do for our health. In the scientific community, an expanding body of research has linked gut health to our wellbeing. We're learning that the trillions of bacteria that live in our gut can interact with our bodies, carrying specific functions which may influence our digestion, immunity, mood and metabolism. The complexity of this relationship has led some people to label our gut bacteria as an organ in its own right. Furthermore, we now know we can affect our microbiota and the health of our gut via the food we eat. In this chapter, we'll take you on a whistlestop tour of your digestive system and look at the science to give you some practical tips for eating for a healthy gut.

Physiology and functions

Your digestive tract runs all the way from your mouth to your bottom, chemically and mechanically breaking down your food into its constituent nutrients and absorbing them along the way. Its work begins even before food enters your mouth; with your body anticipating its arrival and beginning the production of the first digestive juice your meal will encounter; saliva. Once you swallow, food travels slowly through your digestive tract, propelled by muscles contracting and relaxing along the way, in a process called peristalsis. It's a beautifully complex operation, orchestrated by the nervous and hormonal coordination of 10 organs.

The microbiota

The trillions of bacteria lining your large intestine is known as the 'microbiota'. There are so many of these microbes that you have more bacterial cells in your body than human cells![1] Historically, bacteria were always thought of as dirty, disease-causing and dangerous, so through the ages a lot of our focus on wellness has been spent trying to banish bacteria from our bodies – from antibiotics to eat-your-dinner-off-clean toilet seats. However, in the last decade or so we've started to realise that lack of exposure to germs in our environment may suppress the natural development of our immune system and leave us more susceptible to allergies. We've also come to recognise the huge importance of our own community of bugs, with increasing research investigating the microbiome on human health.

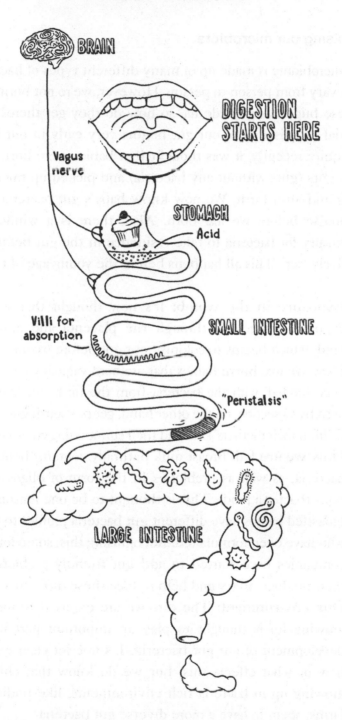

BRAIN

DIGESTION STARTS HERE

Vagus nerve

STOMACH

Acid

Villi for absorption

SMALL INTESTINE

"Peristalsis"

LARGE INTESTINE

Colonising our microbiota

The microbiome is made up of many different types of bacteria, which vary from person to person. However, we're not born with all these bugs living inside us, so how do they get there? The bacterial colonisation of our gut begins very early in our lives. Until quite recently, it was thought that babies were born with sterile guts (guts without any bacteria) and picked up microbes during and after birth. We now know baby's gut bacteria start to colonise before we are born. Also, there is a window of opportunity for bacteria to take residence in the gut before it's effectively 'set'. This all happens before the young age of three.

1) **Exposure in the womb:** It's now thought that we are exposed to bacteria through the placenta and amniotic fluid, which begins to colonise our gut before we are born.[2]

2) **How we are born:** Babies that are born vaginally have their guts 'seeded' with the bacteria from the birth canal. Babies born by C-section, on the other hand, get post-birth gut bacteria from their mothers' skin and their surrounding environment.

3) **How we are fed:** Breast milk naturally contains beneficial bacteria, as well as prebiotics in the form of oligosaccharides (bacteria food). This is thought to be one reason why breastfed babies have different gut bacteria profiles to those who have been formula fed. Recognising this, some formula companies have started to add gut friendly prebiotics to their products to try and help reduce these differences.[3]

4) **Our environment:** The dirt we are exposed to (or not) growing up is thought to play an important part in the development of our gut bacteria. It's not yet clear exactly how or what effects this, but we do know that children growing up in bacteria rich environments, like traditional farms, seem to have a more diverse gut bacteria.

From age three our guts have established their unique profile of bacteria. The next stage is for us to nourish this microbiome with the food we eat to help it thrive.

'Good' and 'bad' bacteria

Bacteria in the gut are often referred to as 'good' or 'bad', depending on how they interact with our bodies. Generally speaking, 'bad' bacteria cause illness or harm to our bodies, whereas 'good' bacteria are the species that not only live alongside us, but promote good health. They help us function at our best by providing us with energy and nutrients, making the environment in our intestine more hostile to bad bacteria, promoting normal immune function and generally keeping our gut healthy. Imbalances, or lower levels of good bacteria, and higher levels of bacteria (known as dysbiosis), have been linked to poor health and an increased risk of diseases like inflammatory bowel disease and diabetes.[4]

Probiotics – is it worth taking them?

The good bacteria we want inside our gut can be found in specialist supplements and food products like yoghurt. The idea is that these products can benefit our health by improving the balance and function of the bacteria in the gut. The balance of gut bacteria might be affected for an array of reasons, including:

- Taking antibiotics.
- Growing older.
- Following gastroenteritis (vomitting and diarrhoea caused by a gut infection).
- Following surgery on the gut.
- Gut illnesses such as IBS or IBD.

Currently there is not enough evidence to recommend taking probiotics if you are already healthy (the science is not quite there yet), but there are some situations where taking a probiotic could be helpful:

1) **Antibiotics:** Antibiotics can play a really important role in fighting off infections. However, they can disrupt the good bacteria as well as the bad, leading one to be prone to getting diarrhoea. Taking probiotics alongside antibiotics (and until a week after) can help protect you from this.

2) **Travellers' diarrhoea:** Commonly known as 'Montezuma's revenge' or 'Delhi belly', it's possible to pick up an infection whilst travelling which causes travellers' diarrhoea. Taking a probiotic containing the bacteria *Saccharomyces boulardii* or a mixture of probiotics called *Lactobacillus acidophilus* and *Bifidobacterium bifidum* for the entire holiday can help reduce the chance of picking up an infection, so you can hopefully enjoy your travels without having to run to the loo unexpectedly.

3) **Treatment of gut disorders:** Probiotics may also play a role in other gut conditions such as IBS (which we'll come to later) and an array of other conditions such as infant colic, vaginal thrush, respiratory tract infections, eczema and food hypersensitivity.[5]

Research has shown that different bacteria in probiotics have different effects on health and disease. This means there is not a standard probiotic which will help with all conditions or symptoms, so it's best to speak with your doctor or dietitian to find one that's right for you. Instead of taking a probiotic supplement it's also possible to get friendly bacteria into your diet by eating fermented foods such as yoghurt, kefir and kombucha.

Prebiotics

Instead of trying to put more friendly bacteria into your gut, you can also try to nourish and increase the amount of those you already have by feeding them with prebiotic foods. These are a type of carbohydrates that survive digestion and manage to make their way to the colon (large intestine) where bacteria feed on them and thrive. Common prebiotic foods are ones that are known to make you a bit windy: onions, garlic, chicory, asparagus, beans and banana.

Talking point: plant diversity

In the past few decades, scientists have started to look at how different foods we eat can affect our gut bacteria. Their research has made one thing at least clear: fibre is key. You'll remember from our carbs chapter that fibre is not digested by our enzymes, so it travels all the way down to the large intestine. It's here that fibre provides food for our gut bacteria, encouraging them to flourish – both in numbers and diversity.

This diversity concept is important. Generally speaking, the more diverse the species of gut bacteria in your gut, the better for your health. This is because different bacteria are involved in different roles and this appears to have an impact on our risk of disease.

When thinking about fibre, we think plants. Interestingly, research published in 2018 implies it's not 'just' about eating plants, but the **number of different** plant foods you eat. A study undertaken by the American Gut Project recruited 10,000

▶

people to provide stool samples and complete food surveys about their diets. They found people who ate 30 different plant foods on a regular basis had a more diverse population of gut bacteria than those who consumed 10 or fewer. The key take-home from this is that you can eat a diet that's good for your gut whether you're a meat-eater or vegan, so long as you consume a large variety of veggies and other plant matter.

Colonic irrigation

Colonic irrigation is a popular trend in the wellness industry. It's claimed that it boosts bowel function, improves the skin and generally makes you feel lighter and brighter. The rationale for its use was based on the 'autointoxication' theory, founded on the belief that toxins residing in the gut can enter the blood, poisoning the body.[6] This became particularly popular in the Western world during the late 1800s, when respected physicians often prescribed it for their patients. Since then though, its use in mainstream medicine has dried up, falling out of fashion in the 1930s when medical professionals refuted the theory of auto-intoxication and criticised the practice. But colonic irrigation is now back, with a new image. Having been rebranded as colonic hydrotherapy (possibly in an attempt to make having a tube stuck up your rectum and your colon swished out with water sound more appealing!), the treatment is popping up in spas and wellness clinics across the country, with colon hygienists even offering hen party packages to get your gut squeaky clean. But despite being touted as a natural way to enhance one's wellbeing and celebrity endorsements, do the claims for this therapy stack up against the science?

Myth busting: colonic irrigation

Dr James Stewart, consultant in gastroenterology

Proponents of colonic irrigation often allude to the fact that it has been practised since the time of the Ancient Egyptians. Whilst this may be true, that does not necessarily mean that it has any proven health benefits. Practitioners of 'colonic hydrotherapy' state that it can improve not only bowel health but general health through the removal of 'toxins' from the large bowel (colon). Is this true?

Historically, medical students were always taught that the purpose of the colon was only to remove water from the stools to make them formed and expel the waste from the body. We now realise that the bowel has many more functions than this and that the bacteria in the bowel are central to gut health.

Colonic irrigation has the potential to remove these 'good bacteria' from the bowel, which may in turn reduce the ability of the microbiome to deliver its important functions. Whilst types of colonic irrigation (enemas) are used in medical practice for conditions such as chronic constipation, and to clear the bowel prior to medical procedures, they are not used for any other purpose and there is no evidence to their benefit beyond this.

Indeed, there is some risk to having a tube inserted into the rectum in the form of rectal perforation (a puncture), and unnecessary cleaning of the bowel can lead to dehydration and electrolyte imbalances. Side-effects are particularly thought to increase if you have a history of gut disease (such as diverticulitis or Crohn's) or a history of kidney and heart disease.[7]

▶

In 2009, researchers reviewed 17 science papers related to colon cleansing and published their findings in the journal *Nature*. They concluded there were no convincing clinical trials or case studies to back up its beneficial claims. They did find, however, numerous reports of serious adverse reactions and complications. Another review in 2011 found most reported adverse effects ranged from vomiting and tummy pain to more serious side-effects such as electrolyte imbalances and kidney failure. A recent case study even reported an event where a gentleman developed septic shock (a life-threatening infection) following a spa session involving colonic irrigation with herb-infused water.[8] Researchers believe the increased pressure on this man's colon caused bacteria to move from his gut into his bladder and blood, leading to the infection. There are also reports of several deaths following 'coffee enemas'.

It's also worth noting that colon-cleansing practitioners are not licensed by a scientifically recognised organisation. 'Therapists' may have undergone training, but the practice is unregulated across the country, despite companies attempting to create their own professional-sounding certifications and regulatory bodies.

In short, despite its long history and current popularity, there is little evidence of benefit and some risks attached to colonic irrigation.

The perfect poo

We often don't like to talk about our toilet habits, but pooping is a vital part of being well. From when we were wee bubs soiling our nappies between one and nine times per day (breastfed babies are at the higher end of the scale), adults on average poop once per day, with most of us passing between three per day to three per week.[9] As you can tell, the amount we poop is a variable pastime and there's definitely no 'normal'. Geography even plays a role, with those in developing countries averaging about two poops per day, possibly because of differences in diet.

Why is this so important? A healthy poop has been linked to lower risks of chronic gut disorders like bowel cancer and constipation.[10] If you think about it, pooing is effectively the removal of waste from the body, so it makes sense that an efficient elimination process should be in place to help get toxins out and keep the gut in tip-top shape.

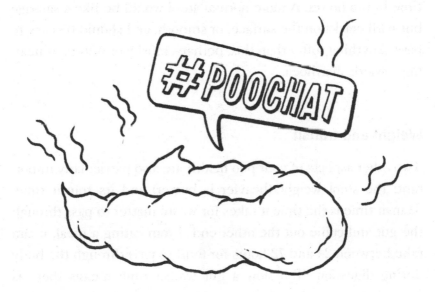

Colour

The brown colour of your poo often isn't just waste from the food you eat, it's some of your body's waste, too. Red blood cells, for example. These blood cells break down into a substance called bilirubin which interacts with a waste product called bile from the liver.

This gives poop its beautiful brown hue. Poos can be other colours, too, and this might be related to the food you eat. Beetroot can turn poop red, liquorice can turn them black and leafy greens can make them green. However, it's always best to speak to your GP if you see anything that's not normal for you. Red or black poop may be caused by bleeding, not food, and pale-yellow poops, which smell bad and are hard to flush, could mean you have an absorption issue.

Texture

Poo texture is another story. A poo in separate hard lumps, like nuts, and which is hard to pass is likely to have spent the longest time in the bowel. A more normal stool would be like a sausage but with cracks on the surface, or smooth, and should be easy to pass. Anything softer than this, perhaps mushy or watery, is nearing towards diarrhoea.

Weight and transit

Two other aspects of your poo health are also particularly important: the stool weight (heavier is better) and its transit time. Transit time is the time it takes for waste matter to pass through the gut and come out the other end. From eating a meal, it can take between 24 and 72 hours for food to pass through the body during digestion. Too slow a gut transit time means there is potentially more time for toxins in the faeces to interact with cells in the gut wall.

There is an inverse association between stool weight and gut transit time, which means that the bulkier your poo, the quicker it moves through your gut. High-fibre diets produce stools that are bulky, soft and able to move through the gut quickly (yay). People who eat traditional diets in developing countries that are rich in fibre have been found to pass soft stools up to four times the weight of those eating a refined Western diet. An old but interesting study compared the stools of teenage boarding-school pupils who ate an institutional Western diet supplemented with cakes and sweets from the school shop, with rural villagers in Uganda who ate an unrefined, high-fibre, traditional diet.[11] The weight of the Ugandan stools were remarkably higher, weighing an average 470g compared to those of the English teenagers, which were on average 110g. Gut transit time was also faster for the Ugandans, being on average 35.7 hours versus 48 hours.

The gut-brain axis

Have you ever heard of the microbes that live inside your intestines being called a second brain, affecting how we think, feel and behave? When we think of nutrition and health, we often consider physical health, rather than mental health. However, research suggests that the relationship between the food we eat and our brain is bi-directional, linking emotional and cognitive centres of the brain with control and function of the gut. This two-way pathway is in part regulated by several complex mechanisms involving the brain, the nervous system, endocrine (hormonal) system, immune system and our gut. Not only does the brain send signals via a communication network to tell the gut how to behave, your gut microbes may also send messages back, telling the brain how to behave.[12]

Researchers are currently investigating how what we eat can affect the types of messages sent between the gut and the brain. So far, there are lots of animal studies showing promising insights into the potential role of diet to mental health. Probiotics, for example, have been found to improve the health of the brain and lower stress levels in mice. Some emerging research in humans has also found that certain pre- and probiotics can lower stress levels and depressive symptoms. These exciting findings mean the bacteria in our gut *might* play a key role in keeping our brain healthy and perhaps could affect conditions such as stress and depression.

Gut food and mood: a tale of two brains

Dr Ruairi Robertson

If a mouse becomes infected by a microbe called *Toxoplasma Gondii*, an intriguing thing happens: it loses its fear of cats. And unfortunately for the mouse, it usually ends up as dinner for the cat. The reason this happens is that *Toxoplasma Gondii* can only replicate inside a cat and therefore it changes the mouse's behaviour in order to reach its final destination. This fascinating fact demonstrates that tiny microbes can affect how mammals think and behave. Amazingly, the microbes that live inside your intestines may also act as a second brain and affect how we humans feel, think and behave, and your diet may play a role in this process.

These two 'brains' (the one in your head and the one in your gut) are physically and biochemically connected in a number of ways. Your gut is physically connected to your brain through 500 million neurons and nerves. Not only does the brain send messages through this communication network to tell the gut how to behave, your gut microbes may also send messages back, telling the brain how to behave.

Your gut and its bacteria also make lots of chemicals that affect brain function. For example, scientists recently discovered that your gut and its bacteria can make many neurotransmitters, the chemicals that make you feel happy,

▶

sad, stressed, excited. None more so than serotonin, nature's antidepressant, 90 per cent of which is made in your gut, less than 10 per cent is made in your brain.

These fascinating new findings suggest that our gut microbes may play an important role in maintaining a healthy brain throughout life and could even affect our stress levels, anxiety or more serious conditions such as dementia.

Having discovered this amazing communication network between our intestines, gut microbes and brains, scientists have begun to examine how our diets affect the messages that are sent within this system. Many studies in animals have shown that certain probiotics (live bacteria that have a specific health benefit) can improve brain health and reduce symptoms of stress in mice. The evidence in humans however is still quite limited. But some studies show that specific prebiotics (fibers that are food for healthy bacteria) and probiotics may reduce levels of the stress hormone cortisol in humans, improve cognitive function and even reduce symptoms of depression.

This research is still very new therefore it's important not to rely on any nutritional supplement for mental health conditions without consulting a doctor.

Can probiotics help with depression?

The link between our gut bugs and the brain is pretty well researched and disruption of this axis is associated with both physical and mental ill health. It makes sense to think that if we enhance our population of good bacteria (via probiotics), this might benefit our brain and mood, too. Studies looking into whether probiotics can have a role to play in mental health are therefore ongoing! Animal studies, for example, have shown probiotics can dampen the effect of the central stress response system (the hypothalamic pituitary adrenal axis), thought to be overactive in depression, and can also increase serotonin levels (the 'happy hormone'). Since these studies are in animals, findings won't necessarily apply to us, too, but they are a really useful starting point to hint at what might go on inside humans. What's even better are human intervention studies. A recent meta-analysis took the results from 10 human studies which compared the use of probiotics versus a placebo on mood.[13] When data was combined for everyone (healthy individuals and those with depression), no significant benefit in mood symptoms was found. The problem is, many of the studies out there are in healthy people, so it's hard for scientists to take results from healthy individuals and apply these to those with depression. It's also difficult to get meaningful results from trials like this when the studies that currently exist use different doses of probiotics and combinations of bacteria strains. To fully answer whether probiotics can meaningfully help people with depression, we need more well-designed studies, which look at the effects of different bacterial strains, specifically in people with clinically diagnosed depression. Most importantly though, if you are thinking of trying probiotics to see if it helps with depression, it's really important that you discuss this with your doctor and take them in addition to your medical therapy (not instead of).

Conditions of the gut

Gut issues are common; everyone experiences them at some point in their lives and it's been estimated that at least 40 per cent of us have at least one digestive complaint at any one time.[14]

That's a lot of upset tummies! Whether it's indigestion, bloating, wind or that stomach bug that had you running to the loo every five minutes on your annual jaunt abroad, we've all been there and it's never pleasant.

Most of these issues can be avoided or remedied with simple lifestyle interventions. However, if you find that your symptoms aren't alleviated by changes to your lifestyle or helped by over-the-counter treatments, you should see your GP.

Red flag symptoms

Certain gut symptoms should never be ignored and should always be taken straight to a doctor. These include:

- A sudden, ongoing change to the pattern of your bowel habits that lasts for more than six weeks.
- Blood in your poo.
- Unintentional and unexplained weight loss.
- Difficulty swallowing.
- Heartburn, indigestion or stomach pain that gets worse over time.[15]

Irritable bowel syndrome

Irritable bowel syndrome (or IBS) is extremely prevalent in the UK: up to one in five adults suffers from it.[16] Unlike coeliac disease, in IBS there's no physical damage to the digestive tract, so if you could look inside yourself with a camera, everything would appear completely normal. However, uncomfortable symptoms such as wind, abdominal pain and discomfort, constipation, diarrhoea (or alternating episodes of both), make it clear that things aren't quite working as they should be. The actual combinations of these symptoms that people experience can vary considerably, but for many they can be highly debilitating and seriously impact their quality of life.

Sadly, there is no cure for IBS and we currently don't know what causes people to develop it. (It's likely to be the combination of numerous genetic, environmental and lifestyle factors.) However, we do know that episodes can be triggered by environmental things like antibiotics, stress, food intolerances and infections. As up to 89 per cent of people report that food is a trigger for their symptoms,[17] dietary support is an important part of the management of IBS.[18] Additionally, as stress can both trigger and exacerbate symptoms, managing busy and stressful lifestyles is also a necessary part of learning to live with this condition.[19]

If you suspect you have irritable bowel syndrome (or any other gut issues), the first port of call should be your GP. Don't self-diagnose – this is an essential step as your doctor will need to rule out other intestinal disorders, such as coeliac disease or inflammatory bowel disease. They can also point you in the direction of dietary support, as pinpointing the dietary trigger of your symptoms on your own can be tricky, with many people ending up on an overly restrictive diet due to random removal of lots of different foods. See our gut issue diagnosis pathway graphic opposite to assess your options more clearly.

Dietary treatment for IBS

Although there are medications that your doctor may prescribe to help you manage your symptoms, dietary advice remains one of the key parts of IBS management. For about 50 per cent of

THE GUT ISSUE DIAGNOSIS PATHWAY

GUT ISSUE SUSPECTED

- constipation
- abdominal pain
- unexpected weight loss
- fatigue
- wind

- signs of malabsorption ie. low iron blood test result
- bloating
- change in bowel habits
- diarrhoea

DON'T SELF-DIAGNOSE KEEP GLUTEN IN YOUR DIET

VISIT YOUR GP FOR A COELIAC DISEASE BLOOD TEST

 IF NEGATIVE

IF POSITIVE

You may have coeliac disease. See a gastroenterologist for a gut biopsy (the gold standard confirmation of coeliac disease)

IBS diagnosis
(this may be after referral to a gastroenterologist to rule out anything else)

1st line:
IBS diet and lifestyle advice

2nd line:
Referral to a LOW FODMAP dietitian

people, simple diet and lifestyle changes can help them control their symptoms of IBS and drastically improve their quality of life.

First-line dietary IBS advice (adapted from NICE guidelines[20])

- Eat your meals at regular times. Erratic meal patterns may exacerbate symptoms.
- Take your time when you're eating. Try sitting down at a table and chewing your food well.
- Ensure you're well hydrated by drinking plenty of fluid (the best way to check this is to aim for pale, straw-coloured urine).
- Restrict tea and coffee to three cups (two mugs) per day.
- Reduce your intake of alcohol and fizzy drinks.
- Limit fresh fruit to three portions per day.
- If symptoms include bloating and wind, consider increasing intake of oats (e.g porridge) and linseeds (up to one tablespoon per day) and limit intake of gas-producing foods such as beans, Brussels sprouts and sugar-free gum.
- If symptoms include constipation, try gradually increasing your fibre intake alongside ensuring you're getting enough fluids. Doing this too quickly could make symptoms worse.
- If symptoms include diarrhoea, keep your fluids up and limit caffeine. You can also try temporarily reducing your intake of high-fibre foods (when your symptoms are bad) as well as cutting back on sugar-free sweets and products containing sorbitol, mannitol and xylitol.

Low-FODMAP diet

For some people, these broad lifestyle changes don't help control their symptoms and they may want to consider trialling a low

FODMAP diet. FODMAP is an acronym that stands for ferment-able, oligosaccharides, disaccharides, monosaccharides and polyols (which is a bit of a mouthful). Essentially, FODMAPs are a group of short-chain carbohydrates that are poorly absorbed and fermented by the bacteria in your gut. Although this is usually a *good* thing, FODMAPs are generally pre-biotics or 'bacteria food' which help to promote a diverse and healthy balance of bacteria in your digestive system, but in some people, they can lead to IBS symptoms.

The presence of poorly absorbed FODMAPs in our large intestine leads to IBS symptoms in the following ways:

- **Gas production:** the fermentation of FODMAPs by bacteria leads to the production of gases like methane and hydrogen, leading to bloating, wind and discomfort/pain. In some people, this can also contribute to constipation.
- **Water movement:** as FODMAPs are very tiny compounds, they can have an osmotic effect in the large intestine, drawing water into the gut. This can lead to diarrhoea in some people.

Low-FODMAP diets (like gluten-free) have become a bit of a trend. The diet itself was developed by a group of Australian scientists known as the Monash group. For a long time prior to low-FODMAP diets, the only way to help people identify specific dietary triggers for their IBS was through trial and error, in a long and arduous elimination diet. Although there was an awareness that certain foods such as milk, dairy and legumes could cause gas and bloating, little was known about what components of these foods cause a problem and what linked them together. In the last 50 years a lot has changed and our knowledge has developed in this area considerably. Over time, it became clear that certain carbohydrates weren't absorbed very well by some people.[21] By the mid-60s, we recognised lactose (milk sugar) malabsorption could cause bloating, gas and diarrhoea, leading to lactose-free diets becoming commonly prescribed in people with IBS (although with limited success). In the 80s, doctors presented a case study of a child who they had been able to prove had diarrhoea caused by fructose malabsorption, with the use of hydrogen breath testing (a test that can detect increases in hydrogen gases produced by bacteria in bowel). Other studies followed which examined the effects of different types of carbohydrate restrictions on gut symptoms like diarrhoea and IBS, and eventually, in 2004, the Monash group in Australia came up with the acronym that tied all these problem compounds together: FODMAP. Since then, scientists have worked systematically to shape and define the diet. They designed studies looking at its efficacy, they compiled food analysis, measuring and defining the levels of FODMAPs in different foods, and validated ways to accurately assess people's intake. This vast body of work has spread across the world, with researchers from Australia, the UK, the US and New Zealand contributing to the knowledge we have today.

Now we have around 10 randomised controlled studies[22] showing that (when supported by a nutrition professional) the low-FODMAP diet is successful in resolving IBS symptoms in 50 to 80 per cent of people with IBS.[23] A recent meta-analysis that pooled the studies on low-FODMAP diets confirmed that current evidence supports the *short-term* use of low-FODMAP diets in the treatment of IBS.[24]

However, it's not all good news. This is a diet that has been designed to be followed for only a short period of time. It's not a 'bloating diet', as some influencers across social media claim, but a temporary medical diet, designed to help people pinpoint their issues and manage their symptoms. Researchers themselves recognised that although the diet was successful in managing the symptoms of IBS of many, long-term restrictions of FODMAPs could potentially cause more harm to our guts (and us) by starving our good bacteria of the food they need to survive. With this in mind, a small study was conducted which looked at the effects of FODMAP restriction on the numbers of bacteria in the gut of 27 people with IBS (and six healthy people) after three weeks on a low-FODMAP diet.[25] They found that despite the intervention being effective at improving IBS symptoms in the treatment group, the average number of good bacteria, like bifidobacteria, which have known health benefits, dropped by around 47 per cent. Bifidobacteria are linked to health benefits like reducing gut infections, and having low levels is also linked with increased pain scores in IBS. In fact, one study found that people who experienced pain had around five times fewer bifidobacteria in their microbiome compared to those without pain, showing the possible links between dysbiosis and symptoms in IBS.[26] Other studies have found similar results, meaning that although low-FODMAP diets are helpful in the short term as a medical treatment for IBS, over the long term they could cause worsening symptoms and potentially poorer gut health. Beware the wellness guru touting this as a long-term cure-all for post-meal bloating (which on its own can be perfectly normal and is not necessarily an indication that something is wrong with your gut). FODMAPs are healthy bacteria food which can help good bacteria in your gut thrive, and as the diet is so restrictive, there is also the chance that over the long term you could become deficient in some nutrients. However, if you have IBS, following a *temporary* low-FODMAP diet with the support of a qualified health professional could help.

If the low FODMAP diet is temporary, how does it work?

The intervention is a three-stage process: FODMAP elimination, FODMAP reintroduction and FODMAP personalisation. The emphasis in treatment is on the reintroduction and personalisation phase, whereby FODMAPs are challenged and your individual tolerance is determined. This is an extremely important part of the FODMAP process. Although people are often reluctant to reintroduce FODMAPs once their symptoms settle in the elimination phase, it allows you to reintroduce some prebiotic foods in a way that helps control your symptoms. In longer-term follow-ups of people who have followed the low-FODMAP process, 61 to 70 per cent of people have found relief of their symptoms a year later, with most tailoring FODMAPs to their individual tolerance and some even completely reintroducing all FODMAPs back into their diet.[27] It can be quite tricky to do alone, but with the help of a nutrition professional you can reduce the FODMAPs in your diet for two to six weeks to give your gut a bit of a rest and try to rebalance other lifestyle factors. Once your symptoms are settled, each type of FODMAP can be 'challenged' individually in a systematic way to see if there are one or two that are problematic for you and also what your threshold is for eating them. It's important to remember that IBS is often triggered by stress, so there is a small chance that if you find this diet super stressful, your symptoms might get worse.

Our favourite low-FODMAP tools

If you are going through the low-FODMAP process, you may find these tools useful and full of credible advice.

Apps
- Food Maestro.
- Monash University FODMAP diet.

Websites
- https://reintroducingfodmaps.com/
- https://alittlebityummy.com

Cookbooks
- *The FODMAP Friendly Kitchen Cookbook* by Emma Hatcher (Yellow Kite, 2017).

Will probiotics help with IBS?

There's a growing interest in using probiotics as part of treatment for IBS. Scientists have noticed that *some* people who have IBS can have an imbalance of bacteria in their guts. In particular, compared to healthy people, those with IBS may have lower levels of bifidobacteria and lactobacillus species (linked with health benefits) and generally less diversity in the gut.[28] Because of this, it's been suggested that probiotics might be a beneficial treatment for people with IBS, one that can help restore balance to the bacteria in the bowel and reduce symptoms.

However, this is a new area of research, complicated by the fact that different strains of bacteria have different health effects, plus probiotics (with the same strains of bacteria) can have different effects in different people. Therefore, it is currently very difficult to make individual recommendations.

However, probiotics are considered safe and if you have IBS you may wish to see if they make a difference for you. If you choose to do so, you need to follow manufacturer's instructions and dosage for a minimum of four weeks to see if the product makes a difference.

Microbiome mapping

With the rising interest in gut health, microbiome mapping (or sending off samples of poo to a stranger in the post) is becoming increasingly popular. These tests 'map' your microbiome – the DNA of your gut bugs – to tell you which types of bacteria you have living in your bowels and how diverse (how many different types you have) they are compared to other people. Sounds exciting, hey? But are these tests worth your time and money, and what can they tell us?

The test themselves are sound. Scientists use a technique called 16s RNA ribosomal sequencing (it's a bit of a mouthful) to determine what the pattern of bacteria in your gut looks like. However, it's currently unclear as to how this knowledge might be useful or practical for people trying to make dietary changes for their health and, in fact, what conclusions can be drawn from them. The science of the microbiome is very new, so there's still a lot we don't know about the effects of different types of bacteria on our health.

Our gut bacteria are a complex ecosystem, with millions of micro-organisms living inside us and impacting our health. In general, it's thought that a more diverse microbiome is better, as different bacteria carry out different jobs and this seems to influence our disease risk. Less diversity has been linked with 'dysbiosis', a term used to describe a loss of diversity, which has been linked with diseases like Crohn's disease and heart disease (although it's still not fully clear whether the disease causes the dysbiosis or if the dysbiosis contributes to the development of the disease). What scientists can agree on at this stage is that it's very unlikely that there is one perfect, optimal pattern of gut bacteria for health and if there is, we don't know what that looks like. It's more likely that healthy gut microbiomes occur along a spectrum and vary from person to person, with the key indicators of a 'healthy biome' being diversity.

In theory, this means that a healthy person could get their biome tested if they want to, to see how diverse their flora is and if their gut is 'healthy'. However, it's important to remember that our gut bacteria can change readily. What we eat and drink, illness, exercise, age and medications can all have an impact on our gut flora and cause variations. Additionally, responses to dietary changes appear to be very individual, having different effects on the microbiota in different people, and we can't currently predict how an individual will respond to a dietary modification.

The current advice for improving diversity is pretty much the same as advice for improving general health. Eat a variety of different plant foods, including fruits, vegetables, legumes and whole grains. Is expensive testing helpful at this stage? Probably not. Can we tell people exactly what to eat to prevent disease based on their microbiome? Not yet.[29]

Talking point: leaky gut

'Leaky gut' has become a buzzword amongst gut health enthusiasts. It's said to cause all sorts of problems from gastric upset to health conditions like diabetes and inflammatory bowel disease. But what is it?

Leaky gut is the term used to describe an increase in the permeability of your gut wall. In some circles, this 'leaky' digestive tract is said to allow unwanted organisms and compounds (namely bacteria and 'toxins') to pass into your body where they can wreak havoc on your health. But some doctors and scientists disagree and claim that leaky gut is not a thing, so is it really a threat to your health?

The truth is, while people can experience an increase in permeability of their gut walls this doesn't necessarily indicate there is an issue with their gut. This is what Registered Dietitian and gut health researcher Dr Megan Rossi had to say on the matter:

'The tight junctions between our intestinal cells open and close all the time in response to diet (e.g. a high-fat meal), exercise (e.g. long-distance running) and medications (such as some pain killers). These triggers tend to have only a short-term

▶

effect but, in some diseases, exposure to a particular allergen (e.g. gluten in people with coeliac disease) has a more sustained effect on the tight junctions. However, if gluten is strictly avoided in people with coeliac disease the problem is resolved. This brings forward the notion that leaky gut is an effect of an underlying disease rather than the cause of disease.'

Current scientific consensus is that while 'leaky gut' can been seen in some circumstances, e.g. people who have a health condition (like coeliac disease), it's also a perfectly normal phenomenon which occurs in healthy people without causing any real issues. It's a symptom, rather than a diagnosis, which in and of itself can be perfectly benign. If you're getting troublesome gut symptoms, speak to your doctor (and remember while diet can play a role in improving gut symptoms in conditions like irritable bowel syndrome, that there are no magic pills, protocols or potions that have been shown to heal a 'leaky gut').

Food-based recommendations for a healthy gut

To nourish your gut:

Eat more

- **Diverse plant foods:** aim to increase the diversity of your plant-based foods (fruits, vegetables, beans, legumes, nuts, seeds) per week.
- **High-fibre foods:** food like garlic, onions, berries, leeks, whole grains, lentils, beans, chickpeas, bananas and avocado all contain prebiotic fibres that are the perfect dinner for your gut microbes.

Switch to

- **Oily fish:** mackerel, tuna, salmon, herring and anchovies are rich in omega-3 fats that are great for your gut bacteria and brain.
- **Fermented foods:** include some plain yoghurt, kefir, sauerkraut or kimchi in your diet. All these foods are all examples of fermented foods that are rich in healthy bacteria called *lactobacilli*.

Eat less

- **Refined grains:** white bread, rice and pasta all lack the fibre that helps to keep your gut healthy.

11

Eating with Allergies and Intolerances

'Could I have a dairy-free, gluten-free, lactose-free, sugar-free latte please? I'm allergic.' Sound familiar? Today it seems as though everyone has some type of food allergy or intolerance. But what's the difference between the two? And are these conditions as common as they appear to be? The distinction between them can be confusing (they both involve food, after all) and they can share similar symptoms. Apart from allergic reactions having obvious life-threatening problems – as evidenced by the tragic death of 15-year-old Natasha Ednan-Laperouse, who died from an allergic reaction after eating a sesame-containing baguette – the distinction matters because removing foods from the diet without good reason (or professional support) can lead to nutritional deficiencies and promote confusion and anxiety around food, leaving you feeling pretty rotten. In this chapter we'll highlight the most common food allergens and investigate food intolerances such as dairy, lactose and gluten. We'll also unpick the complex world of food allergies and intolerances to give you a clear overview of the differences between the two.

Allergy

Allergies are a hot topic in the media, and it's often claimed that the number of people with an allergy or intolerance in Western countries like the UK is rising at a worrying rate.[1] Although allergies can strike at any age, it's estimated that between 5 and 10 per cent of children have an allergy in the UK.[2] It's much harder to estimate what proportion of the adult population have an allergy but it's likely to be less than that in children. Estimates in kids are more accurate as they are based on tests called oral food challenges, whereas self-reported figures in adults are not particularly reliable – and the confusion between allergy and intolerance means that many people think they have an allergy, when they don't. Nevertheless, it's true that hospital admission rates for food anaphylaxis are on the rise, with a reported 615 per cent increase over 20 years to 2012.[3] Additionally, figures from the EU show that the amount of people admitted to hospital with a severe allergic reaction in 2015 was seven times more than in 2005.[4] It's unclear why there has been such an increase, however, theories range from 'the hygiene hypothesis' (which suggests that our decreased exposure to germs means that we are more susceptible to allergies, due to defects in our immune responses) to changes to weaning practices.[5] However, as it stands, nobody really knows why they are increasing.

Food allergies are caused by the immune system, when our normal immune defences (which are usually fighting infections), go off piste and react abnormally to some proteins found in food. These reactions can appear quickly and be life-threatening – think anaphylactic shock – or hours later and be milder in severity, depending on which parts of the immune system are involved.

Different types of food allergy

Food allergies are generally classified as either IgE or non-IgE mediated allergies. IgE-mediated allergies are the ones that tend to come on quickly, recognisable through symptoms like a rash, swelling, breathing difficulties, nausea and vomiting, such as peanut allergy. Although quite rare, it's the IgE-mediated allergy that is associated with anaphylactic shock, a severe whole-body response to an allergen, which can be life-threatening if not treated. Currently, non-IgE mediated allergies aren't understood as well as IgE food allergies, however, they tend to affect the gastrointestinal tract and come on much more slowly (hours and days later versus five to 30 minutes for IgE food allergy). Symptoms can include nausea, diarrhoea and vomiting, but due to their slow onset, the cause of the allergy can be difficult to pinpoint. Additionally, the severity of an allergic reaction can vary both between people and between exposures in the same person. What might be a mild reaction one time could be more severe the next. Typically with allergic reactions, the severity increases with repeat exposure. This is one reason why it's very important to carry your Epipen with you at all times if you have a food allergy.

Let's have a look inside the body to understand allergies in more detail. When protein is digested by the gut it's broken down into its amino-acid building blocks and absorbed by the body into the blood. Now, for most people this part of digestion isn't usually a problem; because the food poses no threat (as food shouldn't), the immune system remains switched off and tolerates the food. However, if there is a breakdown in the wiring of this tolerance system the body may mistakenly see a food as a threat and become 'sensitised' to it. In this situation, immune cells engulf the offending protein and 'decorate' the outside of their cell with special agents which help cells 'remember' the invader next time they encounter it. These agents are called antibodies – IgE antibodies, to be exact. The next time this same food is eaten by the sensitised person, the body will recognise the protein and release inflammatory substances such as histamine to fight it and remove it from the body. Since the IgE antibodies are found in skin, lungs and mucous membranes, the symptoms of this can be itchiness, swelling, streaming eyes, breathlessness and vomiting.

Non-IgE allergies involve the immune system, but not those special IgE agents. They work more slowly and via a different route. These types of allergies tend to affect the gut, such as cow's milk protein allergy.[6] Interestingly, most kids who develop an allergy to eggs, milk, soya and wheat will grow out of it, however, allergies to nuts and seafood (such as peanut allergy, tree nut allergy, shellfish or fish allergy) tend to stick around for life.

List of common allergens

- Cereals containing gluten, including wheat, rye, barley, oats
- Shellfish and lupin molluscs, including prawns, crabs, lobster, crayfish.
- Eggs.
- Fish.
- Peanuts.
- Soya beans.
- Milk.
- Nuts.
- Celery (including celeriac).
- Mustard.
- Sesame.

Food intolerances

Food intolerances, such as to lactose, are way more common than allergies, but they do not involve the immune system. Instead it's a response from your digestive system to food, generally because you either can't digest the food properly or the food irritates the gut lining. Intolerances can be unpleasant and seriously impact quality of life, but they are not life-threatening. This means that although many people with intolerances choose to avoid foods they experience symptoms with, they don't have to be as stringent as those who have allergies. If you have a food intolerance, symptoms such as diarrhoea, fatigue and bloating can occur minutes, hours or days after eating. Some intolerances are well understood (lactose intolerance is due to an insufficiency of the enzyme used to digest it), whereas many others are not, making them very difficult to diagnose and treat.

List of common food intolerances

- Lactose.
- FODMAPs (see previous chapter).
- Gluten.
- Histamine.
- Salicylates (a natural chemical made by plants such as fruits and vegetables).
- Wheat.
- Sulphur dioxide/sulphites (used as a preservative in dried fruit).

In summary

A food allergy is:

- An abnormal response from the immune system.
- Tends to come on quickly.
- Can be life-threatening.
- Happens every time the food is eaten, even in small amounts.

A food intolerance is:

- Not driven by the immune system.
- Tends to come on gradually.
- Symptoms can relate to the amount and frequency of food.
- Is not life-threatening.

Talking point: gluten intolerance – is it a thing?

We'd like to talk about gluten, something many people try to cut out of their diet, due to fears about its effects. It's true that some people can't eat gluten for medical reasons, but how many people who remove gluten really know why they're cutting it out? Or what gluten even is?! The American chat-show host Jimmy Kimmel decided once to put this question to the public by sending out his camera crew to ask gluten-free members of the public in LA a simple question: 'What is gluten?' Responses included: 'This is pretty sad, cos I don't know', 'It's like a grain, right?', 'I haven't researched it to the fullest. I have a girlfriend

▶

from Russia, she just got me into it, so she's writing a book about it', and 'It's the part, I believe, of the wheat that . . . I really don't know!' This exercise highlighted how health trends drive people to willingly restrict foods without understanding why.

From a medical perspective, the people who need to avoid gluten completely are those with a condition called coeliac disease. Coeliac disease is a common digestive disorder which is estimated to affect around one in 100 people in the UK. When people with coeliac disease consume gluten, their guts become inflamed and unable to absorb nutrients. This can lead to nutrient deficiencies and, over the long term, health problems like osteoporosis. The only treatment we have for this is a lifelong gluten-free diet.

What exactly is gluten? Gluten is a family of proteins found in grains such as wheat, rye and barley. The two main proteins in the gluten family are called glutenin and gliadin. These proteins cause damage to your small intestine by triggering an immune reaction, causing the immune system to attack the lining of the gut.

Coeliac disease can be pretty hard to spot. In fact, it's been estimated that around 500,000 people in the UK have undiagnosed coeliac disease. One reason for this is that the symptoms can be pretty variable and many people don't experience any symptoms at all. However, the most frequent symptoms when they do occur are tummy pain, cramping or bloating, diarrhoea, fatigue, nausea or vomiting and weight loss, which means it can often be mistaken for other gastro disorders, such as irritable bowel syndrome. If you suspect you have coeliac disease, it's really important you go to your GP to get tested. However, it's also really important that you don't

▶

cut out gluten until you have a diagnosis. This might sound counterintuitive, but because the methods used to detect coeliac disease depend on the presence of gluten in your diet, excluding it before a test can mean that it comes back negative, even if you have the condition.

Non-coeliac gluten sensitivity

While those with coeliac disease must avoid gluten to prevent the immune system attacking the lining of their gut, there may be a group of people (estimated 0.5–13 per cent[7]) with a condition dubbed non-coeliac gluten sensitivity. This condition was first so-named in 1978 when a patient without coeliac disease found their gut issues improved after following a gluten-free diet.[8] Some researchers question whether this condition actually exists, while others think it's possible that people who believe themselves to be gluten intolerant are sensitive to something else in food. A recent well-designed, randomised controlled trial tested this theory, by feeding people with self-reported non-coeliac gluten sensitivity muesli bars.[9] In these bars were either hidden gluten, fructans (a type of poorly digested, fermentable carbohydrate) or a placebo bar with neither ingredient. The scientists found that, on average, there was no difference in the symptoms between the people eating gluten and a placebo. However, interestingly, the group eating fructans had significantly more symptoms than the other two groups, supporting the theory that NCGS may be a form of irritable bowel syndrome.[10] For now, this means that the condition remains a contentious topic amongst scientists, but more research is being carried out which will hopefully expand our understanding of this area and lead to more answers for people who have this problem.[11]

Allergy testing

Unfortunately there isn't one single test that can diagnose a food allergy or intolerance by itself. It's complex stuff and even the invasive blood tests can get it wrong, with potential false positives and negatives. Food intolerances are easy to confuse with allergies and self-diagnosis is all too common. This leads people to worry about things unnecessarily, potentially cutting out food groups or following the wrong treatment.

Allergies involve antibodies, they don't always involve symptoms. This means that in order to diagnose allergies, antibodies must be tested for and it's possible someone could have allergic symptoms but not actually have an allergy. Adverse reactions to food might be an intolerance (think headache, wheezing, racing heart, coughs or hives).

If you suspect you have a food allergy or intolerance, you'll need a face-to-face consultation with your GP, a specialist doctor (such as a clinical immunologist) or dietitian to go through some, or all, of the following: your symptom history, a skin-prick test or specific IgE blood test if an allergy is suspected (measuring IgE antibodies in response to an allergen) and a food exclusion diet + challenge.

Do home intolerance tests work?

The use of complementary and alternative medicines to diagnose food allergy and intolerances is growing fast. There are so many types of 'tests' available on the high street and it's very hard to know what's reliable and evidence-based. Kinesiology, hair analysis and pulse tests all sound very exciting, but the science behind their efficacy is poor. This means people are subject to being misdiagnosed and potentially following a poor diet due to unnecessary food exclusions. Although there's talk about allergies being on the rise in the Western world, it's possible numbers are being skewed by the 'worried-well' receiving false diagnoses. In fact, only about 1–2 per cent of the UK have diagnosed food allergies. It's becoming increasingly common for people to use home testing kits to try to diagnose a food allergy or intolerance. These kits are widely available in shops and online and it can be really hard to know if they're reliable. Most online food intolerance 'tests' (e.g. the Hemocode or York Test) involve something called IgG testing. These widely advertised tests analyse the blood IgG antibodies produced in response to eating different foods. They claim an increase in IgG antibodies to a specific food – such as eggs – means you're intolerant to it. The trouble is, these tests appear to be legitimate, when they aren't. Journalist Alex Gazzola, who specialises in allergies and food intolerances, told us: 'Those who've had personal success with IgG and then evangelise about it, can be dangerously and plausibly convincing.'

But this is far from the truth. Let's see what the experts say.

Believe it or not, the production of IgG antibodies is just *a normal and healthy response to eating food*.[12] [13] It's actually 'a measure of exposure' (aka a sign that you've eaten that food recently). Put simply, having IgG antibodies in your blood for a particular food stuff is your body's way of saying: 'I can see you've eaten that food and it's been tagged', not 'you're intolerant to that food'. And, in fact, having IgG antibodies in the blood is a sign that your body is tolerant to the food – something that's protecting us! Despite many experts attempting to debunk IgG testing in the public domain, they are still promoted and sold. 'So how do we effect change?' queries Gazzola. Hair analysis tests and kinesiology are also unproven methods that have no scientific basis to diagnose intolerances. It's the bad science underpinning these two tests that Gazzola thinks should be tackled first, 'being far easier to prove as 100 per cent nonsense'.

Are IgG tests useful at all? Not for diagnosing allergies or food intolerances; in fact, there are currently no reliable and validated clinical tests for the general diagnosis of food intolerances yet. You might feel you want a 'quick fix', but these online tests are often misleading, wasting your money, time and potentially jeopardising your health. There is the risk that invalid tests would recommend you inappropriately restrict your diet or seek potentially harmful treatment.

Immunologists are increasingly seeing parents who, in good faith, have removed foods out of their children's diets due to an 'allergy' based on these 'tests' (which have no scientific backing), putting them at an increased risk of nutritional deficiency.

Debunking complementary therapy allergy tests

IgG

The claim: to identify food intolerances via finger-prick blood testing and IgG analysis.

Expert consensus: IgG antibodies are a marker of exposure to a food, not a marker of intolerance or allergy. Presence of an IgG antibody for a food just tells you that you ate it recently. It may be more of an indication of tolerance than intolerance.

Kinesiology

The claim: changes in energy fields can be detected through muscle weaknesses when people are exposed to vials that contain the essence of certain foods which are placed on the body. A muscle weakness indicates an intolerance.

Expert consensus: there is no evidence that this practice works – like many of these tests, it lacks scientific rationale.

Hair analysis

The claim: testing hair for minerals can indicate food intolerances.

Expert consensus: the actual way these tests are carried out is not very clear, nor is how this would link to allergies or intolerances. There's no evidence to support its use and this kind of testing is a waste of money.

Electrodermal (Vega) test

The claim: an electro-acupuncture-type device measures changes in skin conductivity or 'energy levels' when the patient is exposed to a potential allergen.

Expert consensus: this test has no established scientific grounding and there are no controlled trials to support its claims.[14]

Recommended resources

If you think you may have an allergy or intolerance or just want to find out more, www.allergyuk.org has credible information. They also have a helpline with free access to allergy specialist dietitians and a chat messaging system to talk through concerns.

Read the guide to what allergies are (and aren't) and the evidence for causes and treatments at Sense about Science: Making Sense of Allergies PDF.[15]

12

Diet Culture
and Weight Stigma

Whether we buy into it or not, weight, health and beauty are often inseparable in our minds. From the beauty ideals enforced by the media to the government health messaging that places blame and responsibility firmly on individuals, our bodies have become not only a vehicle for our daily lives but a signal to society of our discipline, intelligence, wealth and even moral fibre.

In times gone by, if you weren't considered particularly attractive (by conventional standards), you basically had to accept it and get on with living your life, focusing on the stuff you enjoyed and that was important to you. But those heady days are long gone, now we're sold this idea that if you're not quite 'hot' enough yet, there is plenty to buy, do and worry over in order to remedy the matter. Even subliminally, the suggestion is everywhere: the idea that we should starve, cut, mould, shape and abuse our bodies in our quest for the holy grail of hotness. There are a zillion ways you can 'fix' your body: you can eat next-to-nothing on a super-low-calorie diet or, if that doesn't make you miserable enough, you could pay thousands of pounds for a wellness retreat, paying for the privilege of fasting yourself to glory in the remote Alps (where nobody can hear you scream). You can have hair extensions, teeth whitening, botox, liposuction, facelifts and lip fillers. You can hire a personal trainer to HIIT your fat away, build abs and finally become the thin, gorgeous you that you always knew you could be. And then – so the line of thinking goes – everybody will love you. If you want, you can even buy the hair products that those new-fangled CGI 'faux-influencers' use to make their hair so shiny. Wait. What?

This is diet culture.

Diet culture is not easy to define, but in its simplest sense it's a system of beliefs and values which reinforce the idea that our bodies, and by extension ourselves, aren't 'good' enough or beautiful enough as they are, and therefore need to be fixed. Unfortunately for us, the insidiousness of diet culture lies in the fact that it's rooted so deeply within us and it's so widespread that it can be hard to pinpoint precisely. It's sneaky like that. It exists within the promise that you can lose weight quickly, easily and permanently and that the only thing stopping you is yourself. It's there in all the implicit and explicit marketing of foods and regimens that promise to make you thinner. It's diet culture that tells you to ignore your growling stomach and lightheadedness in the face of extreme hunger and that sells us zero-calorie faux noodles that will expand in our stomach and fill us up, without providing any actual sustenance for our body. And, crucially, it's there in the fundamental belief that your body is something to be viewed and judged, rather than a means through which you live your life. It's all these things, and so much more, a shifting illusion of perfection which pops up everywhere, sometimes even dressed up as antidotal, non-diet messages. Diet culture, it turns out, is a bit of a bitch. It's the antithesis of diversity. A covert operation designed to convince us that pushing all our energy and cash into changing our appearance is an important and worthwhile pastime.

Unsurprisingly, something's got to give. It's currently estimated that around 60 per cent of adults in the UK are ashamed
of the way they look.[1] Girls as young as five years old have
expressed concerns about their appearance, with one in five
primary school girls reporting that they have been on a diet.[2] A
recent survey also found that after watching reality TV shows
like *Love Island*, around 21 per cent of 18 to 24-year-olds felt
they were more likely to consider having plastic surgery.[3] This
is big business; globally, the diet and fitness industries combined are estimated to be worth a staggering £125 billion (and
rising), making money through their diet plans, transformation
programmes and weight-loss clubs. Non-invasive cosmetic
surgeons and illegal drug providers appear to have benefitted
from our narrowing definitions of beauty, too. Steroid use in
young men is thought to have quadrupled between 2015 and
2016 and the number of people undergoing non-invasive procedures like lip fillers and botox has skyrocketed, reflecting
both the pressures to conform to certain standards and also the
increasing acceptance of these treatments as a 'normal' part of
a beauty regime.[4]

This growing market for cosmetic procedures is interesting, given the shift in the way we now approach diets. 'Diets!
Nobody does that anymore!' I hear you say. And you're right:
despite their wild popularity in the 80s, we're decades past the
age where everybody and their dog was proudly on a diet of
some description. Now, it's not cool to diet. You still need to be
thin, but socially it's bit more complex. You can't admit to being
on a diet (too tryhard). No. Thinness must be *effortless* and it also
must be healthy. Following a diet is naff. Except, when you don't
call it a diet.

Modern-day dieting is just more evolved than the regimes
of the past. We don't 'South Beach' or 'Atkins' anymore, now
we choose a lifestyle, we wear our eating regimes like a fashion

accessory, a signal to our peers that we're part of the tribe and we care about our health and our body. These lifestyles promise us the earth. They make the complex simple. Find your tribe, follow the rules, you'll be thin, beautiful, stave off disease; they promise you health, happiness and, most importantly, Life. The darker, less obvious side to this is the sinister, unspoken threat: don't do these things and you'll get fat. You'll get the disease. You'll die.

Naturally, the perceived healthfulness and success of these 'lifestyles' is all tied up with the way people look. We see the young, slim and stylish wellness blogger as a walking testimonial for how fantastic her food choices and lifestyle are for her health. People we consider to look 'healthy' (some cynics would say this is a euphemism for thin) are assumed to have made superior choices, have more self-discipline and be more morally sound. And of course the reverse is true as well; we're encouraged to automatically associate excess weight with a series of profoundly damning personality traits. Do you see the problem here?

We see all this as a worrying trend towards a brand new 'ism': 'healthism'. The idea that health is a moral responsibility, resulting in an unparalleled focus on health and the belief that poor health is a personal failing. Healthism fails to consider the complexities of each individual body, genetically as well as socially and economically, putting the emphasis firmly on individual responsibility. Inevitably, diet culture's in the driving seat, and unsurprisingly this quest for the perfect diet, the perfect body and the perfect life has had some less-than-healthy consequences for some people. A prominent and growing diagnosis is orthorexia, an unhealthy obsession with health and perfection or purity, pursued to such an extent that it becomes detrimental to your health.

In pursuit of perfection

Type #Fitspo (or to give it its full and proper title, 'fitspiration') into Instagram and your device will direct you to millions of photos (54.4 million at the time of writing), largely featuring poised, lean, 'ideal' bodies, celebrating thigh gaps, ab cracks and the 'peach' (a round, gravity-defying bum).[5]

Just to put fitspiration into perspective, let's look at its origins: the widely shared term is the fitness industry's take on the pro-anorexia buzzword '#thinspiration' – a trend that sees images of ultra-thin women posted online to inspire others and to encourage deeply disordered eating patterns. Fitspiration, on the other hand, encourages people to exercise in the pursuit of lean, muscular 'fit' bodies. (See also #strongnotskinny.) Despite fitspo's ostensibly healthier outlook and good intentions, it still has the same idea at its heart: that images of bodies should be used to motivate people to participate in certain behaviours. Studies investigating the effects of images and messages about health which induce feelings of shame have shown us that people who feel badly about their bodies are less likely to take care of them, not more.

Research into the fitspiration movement has also revealed some concerning issues.[6] A comparison of content revealed that the images and messages shared are strikingly similar to those posted by people promoting 'thinspiration', its more sinister cousin. On analysing a random selection of thinspo and fitspo images online, one study found that although the thinspo sites featured more content praising thinness or providing food-guilt messages, both were equally culpable when it came to weight stigmatisation and messages advocating restrictive dieting practices. This, and other research like it, has indicated that although thinspiration websites are widely known to contain potentially damaging material, other online platforms supposedly devoted to healthy pursuits could contain content along worryingly similar themes.

If 'aspirational' is something desirable and lusted after, and 'inspirational' is something that might spur you into action, where does fitspo fall? Or put another way, does setting up somebody else's body as a '#goals' motivate people to exercise more or eat better? Turns out, probably not. And science agrees.

Most images related to the fitspiration hashtag are of ideal bodies either posing or exercising, sometimes with quotes attached to them like, 'you don't get the ass you want by sitting on it' (nice). We know that exposure to aspirational bodies, particularly amongst women, drives us into the comparison trap, i.e. it promotes body dissatisfaction, encouraging us to objectify our own bodies and think about our 'flaws'. Body dissatisfaction is not healthy; it's been linked with increased risk for anxiety, depression and eating disorders.[7] We also know that people who feel dissatisfied with their bodies are less likely to take care of them and more likely to engage in risky behaviours.[8][9] On the flip side, people who accept and love their bodies are more likely to move them and to eat well. One recent example of this was shown in a collection of studies which examined[10] the effects of two fitness campaigns aimed at women: the UK's 'This Girl Can' campaign and the Australian #jointhemovement campaign, both of which focused on showcasing a diverse range of bodies engaging in and enjoying exercise in a realistic, non-idealised style. These studies examined the effects on women of viewing these 'real' campaigns versus idealised 'fitspiration' images, with a particular focus on how they made them feel about their own bodies and how motivated they felt to go and exercise. They showed, unsurprisingly, that campaigns that include a range of body shapes and sizes, as well as people from a variety of ethnicities, cultures and backgrounds, made women feel better and more satisfied with their own appearance (i.e. they promoted body positivity) and led to increased motivation to exercise. They also showed that while campaigns like this can't protect us from the negative effects of the barrage of sculpted, photoshopped bodies in the media (women who subsequently viewed the fitspiration images were still drawn into the comparison trap), seeing a true reflection of diversity, including people we look like exercising, makes a message more inspirational than aspirational. With this in mind you can see why, for us, examples of diversity in sport, like Jada Sezer and Bryony Gordon's decision to run the 2018 London Marathon in their underwear was infinitely more inspiring – to exercise and improve your health at any size – than any 20-something fitness blogger posing online in their gym gear.

So perhaps fitspiration has more insidious consequences for our physical and mental health than we might expect. But the people with washboard abs posting these photos must be healthy, right?

Well maybe. But it's certainly not a guarantee.

Getting a six-pack isn't easy: you have to be *lean*. This may not be difficult for some people (especially if it's their job), but for most it requires meal planning and prepping, restricting intake or dieting, committing large amounts of time to a tailored training plan, and prioritising it over and above other things. For some people this may be doable, but for many others, the sacrifices involved in maintaining this lifestyle and the restrictions they would be placing on themselves in order to try to mimic the muscle they see online would prove deeply unsustainable and potentially play havoc with both their physical and mental health. In all of this, it's crucial to remember that what we venerate as 'the perfect body' may not align with what is healthy for our own bodies. We are not all designed to look the same. This is especially true for women, where we know that very low body fat percentages, coupled with high exercise demands and restrictive diets can cause demonstrable physical problems, with some women temporarily losing their periods – something called hypothalamic amenorrhoea. It's something of a taboo in women's fitness (and some girls think nothing of it), but intensive fat-loss programmes like the ones followed by figure competitors and people trying to 'cut' fat from their bodies, have long been linked with period irregularities, giving rise to concerns that the focus on 'leanness' as a beauty standard is putting more women at risk of their menstrual cycles stopping and suffering the subsequent issues that come with low oestrogen levels, including an increased risk of osteoporosis.

The unintended consequence of our obsession with weight: weight stigma

Diet culture feeds stereotypical negative beliefs about fat bodies (we use fat here in the fat-positive, reappropriated sense), portraying them as lazy, weak-willed, unattractive, unfit and greedy, which in turn perpetuates weight stigma.[11][12] Weight stigma is the umbrella term for the negative perception of fat people and the attitudes that are directed towards them. People can experience weight stigma through daily microaggressions (think people rolling their eyes at you or tutting) and through explicit verbal or physical abuse for simply being in their body. Let's be clear: weight stigma is a form of discrimination, which people in larger bodies experience as a result of our entrenched attitude that fatness is a personal responsibility and moral issue, rather than an outcome influenced by a complex mix of physiological, biological, environmental and social factors.

Even amongst healthcare professionals, it's common to think that shame or fear can be a good motivator for health improvement[13][14], but weight stigma research paints a very different picture.

Far from being a driver for positive change, many studies show that experiencing weight stigma increases the likelihood of you engaging in risky behaviours such as reduced physical activity.

Think about it: how often would you want to go for a walk or a run outside if every time you did strangers eyeballed you with disdain or made jokes at your expense? Studies in children have shown that those who experience weight-related teasing (even if they aren't categorised by medical standards as overweight) are much more likely to display signs of disordered eating and participate in unhealthy weight-control practices, like extreme food restriction, and much less likely to participate in physical activity.[15]

As well as risky behaviour, weight stigma has also been linked with both psychological and physiological poor health. By this we mean it's been linked with an increased risk of diabetes, disordered eating, depression, anxiety, body dissatisfaction and ... wait for it ... weight gain.[16] And despite the best intentions of healthcare providers, negative attitudes held towards those in larger bodies can impact on the quality of the care they provide. Research has shown such attitudes can affect that healthcare provider's behaviour and decision making.[17] A referral to a physio may be refused for a non-weight-related injury, a weight-loss diet may be suggested instead of further investigation into fatigue and there are even accounts online of cancer diagnoses being delayed or missed by doctors unable to see past someone's size. These are weight biases, one's own internalised attitudes and beliefs about weight which are influenced heavily by our own culture and experiences. And they seem to have already been formed when healthcare professionals are students, with one UK study finding 'unacceptable levels' of weight bias and fat phobia among trainee nurses, doctors, nutritionists and dietitians.[18]

So far this is a relatively new area of research. Indirectly, weight stigma is thought to negatively impact on those in larger bodies by making them less likely to stick to a medical plan or avoid seeking medical help in the first place. It's currently not clear if weight stigma directly causes poor health conditions, although there are some studies that show how it could cause physical harm, through its effects on the stress hormone cortisol, increased inflammation and other metabolic derangements.[19] [20] Weight is not a lifestyle choice or behaviour, it's an outcome that is influenced by genetics, social and environmental factors (to be extremely simplistic). This is an assumption (bias) that leads people to believe others are 'to blame' for their weight, so shame is justified. But as it stands, all signs point to this; shaming people does not improve their health and it may well be harmful.

We should say here that challenging internal bias or beliefs can be tough. The first rule of bias club, they say, is that you don't know you're in bias club after all. The beliefs we have about fatness and fat bodies are often subconscious and reinforced by the culture we live in. Interestingly, in addition to this, although most weight stigma is experienced by people in large bodies, the effects have also been shown in some studies to be independent of weight, meaning that even people of a 'normal' body mass index who 'think' that they are overweight or obese may experience its negative effects – diet culture is messing with all of us, and it needs to stop. So how can we fight diet culture? By breaking up with diets and weight talk.

Breaking up with diets and weight talk

'Have you forgotten about obesity?' we hear you cry. 'We have a war on our hands, a full-blown crisis! AN EPIDEMIC! We need diets because people are so fat! People can't just eat what they want!' Well that's the diet culture talking, folks. Letting go of all that rubbish does not mean 'letting yourself go'. Stopping playing the diet culture game isn't something many of us can just do (more on that in a moment) but turning your back on the part of our culture designed to make you feel that you aren't healthy/happy/beautiful enough as you are is one of the healthiest, most liberating things that you can do. Diet culture has taught us that we can't trust our bodies. We need food-recording apps, meal plans, dietary restrictions, rules and nutrition professionals in place to control ourselves around food and to keep ourselves healthy. And in some ways, this is true. Diets or, more specifically, rules, can be the thing that help us to comfortably navigate eating in the real world, that help us to keep our fears at bay – whether that be fear of weight gain, illness or death. In some cases, the structure and consistent framework of a particular diet can be the life-raft that keeps people afloat in a stressful wider eating culture. But as we discussed in the calories chapter, restriction and dieting doesn't necessarily lead to healthier (or lighter) bodies. Unpicking our relationship with these doctrines and lifestyles can be complex and time-consuming (and it's not necessary for everyone), but if your interactions with food are fraught with anxiety and guilt, or your relationship with food occupies too much of your head space, it might just be time to break up with diets and diet culture.

Why break up with diets?

Breaking up with diets doesn't mean breaking up with healthy behaviours like eating well and exercising. The difference is your mindset. Instead of doing these things to lose weight, which might involve following a punishing exercise routine that you dread or a strict meal plan that leaves you feeling hungry (and guilty when you inevitably face-plant into a packet of biscuits), you find a way to eat and move your body that you enjoy and which makes you feel good. It's the ultimate in self-care. And that's a lifestyle (not a diet).

▶

Dieting may be negatively impacting on your health if:

- Your diet is causing you to feel anxious or low in mood.
- You are locked in a cycle of weight loss/weight gain (and weigh more now than you did when you started dieting).
- You feel shame about your body and past dieting failures.
- You are preoccupied with food.
- You have found yourself in a cycle of restrict/binge (aka you diet then get so hungry you eat everything in sight).
- You think you need to lose weight, but people around you don't agree.

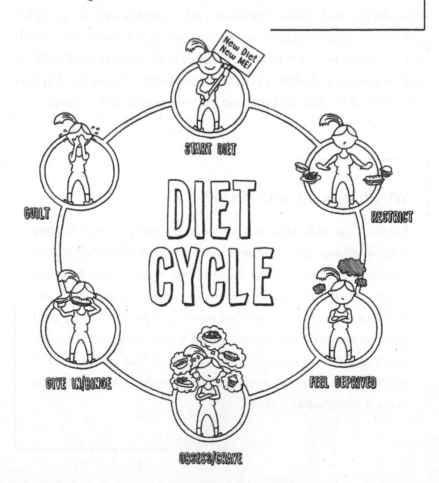

When it comes down to it, taking pride in your body and health doesn't mean aspiring to a certain shape or size. Exercise doesn't need to be tied to aesthetics either. What about exercising for fun? Because you love your body? Because it makes you feel good? Because you know it will benefit your health? The benefits of exercise go way beyond abs. Let's not forget that despite good intentions, the images dominating the #fitspo news cycle can make health seem completely out of reach for many people. So if you're happy and you want to focus on your diet and sculpt your body, that is totally up to you – no judgement from us. But remember that there's no 'right' way to have a body, and healthy bodies come in all different shapes and sizes. Exercising and eating well is something we can all strive for, no matter what our size.

So if not diets, then what?

Something that has been a little lost in the conversation around diets in Western culture is the idea that we can place trust in our bodies and ourselves to know how and what to eat. We're obsessed with outsourcing to meal plans and asking experts 'is this good for me?' and 'should I be eating this?' Intuitive eating is a philosophy of eating which puts you back in the driver's seat when it comes to your body and its hunger signals. It's about focusing our attention on 'how' to eat rather than 'what' to eat, taking the emphasis away from what the body looks like and putting it back on how the body feels. The process itself was created by two pioneering American dietitians – Evelyn Tribole and Elyse Resch – whose book *Intuitive Eating* still provides the blueprint for the dietary intervention today. Essentially, eating intuitively is the opposite of a traditional diet (hurrah!) as it does not impose guidelines about what or how to eat. Instead, it teaches us to enjoy food, honour our hunger or fullness signals and respect our body. All foods can fit within a healthy diet and intuitive eating recognises that, placing them all on a level playing field, taking away the food hierarchy which categorises foods as 'good' or 'bad' (and consequently implies that you are good or bad as a result of your dietary choices). While it's still a relatively new and exciting area of nutrition research, studies have shown us that this approach could be useful not only for building a healthier, more balanced relationship with food, but also for improving your health and your body image.[21] [22]

A 2014 systematic review of 26 studies found that intuitive eaters were more likely to have lower body weights, healthier eating behaviours and better mental health.[23] Some of the experimental studies (randomised controlled trials) included in this review also showed that people who underwent intuitive eating counselling had improved markers of physical health – from cholesterol to blood pressure and inflammation – compared to other interventions (e.g. a weight-loss group). In one study with longer-term follow-up, cholesterol remained significantly improved from its baseline measures at the start of the study. That said, we are waiting for further studies with more diverse participants and extended follow-ups before any firm conclusions can be drawn about its universal application. What we do know now is that it has proved quite effective in young women, especially those who have a troubled relationship with food.

One of the problems with intuitive eating is that it's widely misunderstood. The phrase is often thrown around casually on social media by self-styled gurus telling us to 'just listen to our body' or 'eat intuitively', without any information about how to do this in practice. Learning how to eat intuitively is a complex process which takes time, patience and self-understanding. And it isn't for everybody; not everyone has a bad relationship with food. But the *philosophy* of intuitive eating – the essence of it and the principles – holds something for all of us. So far research has linked intuitive eating with healthier relationships with food, lower risk of disordered eating behaviours, lower body mass index and better weight maintenance.[24] Additionally, this way of eating has been shown to be sustainable in the long term (in contrast to most diets), to improve self-esteem, body image and overall quality of life. We don't yet know much about the application of intuitive eating in people with health conditions such as diabetes, so if you need to follow a specific diet for medical reasons, it's important to speak to your doctor or dietitian to discuss the potential risks.

The highs and lows of intuitive eating

Dr Laura Thomas, registered nutritionist and author of *Just Eat It*

Most of us have been on some sort of a diet for as long as we can remember; even when we're not on an 'official' diet, the chances are we've been avoiding foods we really enjoy, or aren't eating as much as we really need to feel satisfied. This can lead us into a cycle of restriction and binging or can cause us to feel anxious or stressed about eating in social situations or around particular foods. Learning about intuitive eating can feel incredibly exciting and liberating (which it is!). However, something I see clinically is that people are so fed up of dieting that they want to race through all the principles of intuitive eating and get to the end without giving the principles a chance to fully sink in.

People are so excited about becoming an intuitive eater that they forget there's a lot of work that has to go into undoing diet rules and *relearning* how to eat; you don't go from

▶

stopping a diet one day to suddenly becoming an intuitive eater the next – it's an active process!

But remember, there's no certificate or medal at the end, so *slow down* and *enjoy it*. Be curious! What happens when you allow yourself to eat the foods you really desire? What happens when you tune into the signals your body is sending you? How does it feel to eat the things that are satisfying as well as nourishing? It won't be perfect; there is no such thing as being a perfect eater, but if you pay attention in a non-judgemental way, like a scientist gathering data, you'll soon discover what feels good in your body rather than being guided by external rules and restrictions; how much food is too little, too much and just right! Which foods give you stamina and a sense of wellbeing, and which foods you eat just because they taste good!

Remember that it can take time to tune back into a way of eating that is best for your body. It can certainly be difficult to let go of a perceived sense of control, but remind yourself that diets and food rules only seem as though they offer control and often come at a high price (like stress or guilt around food). Our bodies don't need to be micromanaged; the process of intuitive eating can help us get out of our heads when it comes to food and eating, and let our bodies call the shots.

Ultimately, cultivating a healthy relationship with food is like cultivating healthy relationships with people. It takes work, it's sometimes difficult or strained, and we are all different, so no two relationships look the same.

As an introduction, here's a short overview of the 10 principles that shape the intuitive eating process.

Ten principles of intuitive eating

1) **Reject the diet mentality:** this principle is based around ditching diet culture and the idea that you need externally imposed rules to regulate your eating.

2) **Honour your hunger:** give yourself permission to respond to your hunger and move away from eating patterns that drive primal hunger and binge eating.

3) **Make peace with food:** by giving yourself permission to eat all foods, even the ones you deem 'bad', you can start to rebuild trust with both food and yourself.

4) **Challenge the food police:** this principle aims to make you aware of and challenge your internal dialogue about food. This involves recognising different internal voices that help or harm your relationship with food, so that you can gradually learn to view food more neutrally.

5) **Feel your fullness:** one of the potential side-effects of chronic dieting is losing the ability to know when you are hungry and when you are full. This principle works to reconnect you with your hunger cues.

6) **Discover the satisfaction:** when we view food exclusively as fuel, or even as the enemy in our pursuit of weight loss, we can lose the joy of eating. This principle is focused on helping people recapture the joy in eating and how to eat mindfully.

7) **Cope with your emotions without using food:** if emotional hunger is your primary coping mechanism, it's likely to have a negative effect in the long run. By focusing on how to meet your needs without food, you can expand your coping repertoire and stop relying on food as the only way to get you through difficult times.

8) **Respect your body:** unpicking unrealistic beauty standards and accepting your body is an essential part of the intuitive

eating process. Developing respect for your body throws into sharp relief the harm you are doing when you punish it for eating or not fitting into certain clothes, or by 'body bashing' with negative body talk.

9) **Exercise – feel the difference:** reconnecting with your body and learning to move in a way you enjoy and which feels good, as well as all the other health benefits that come with exercise (apart from weight loss), is a step towards taking care of your body long term, on its own terms.

10) **Honour your health – gentle nutrition:** the final step in the IE process is gentle nutrition. This final stage acknowledges that there is no such thing as the 'perfect' diet and helps people work towards honouring themselves with foods that nourish both their bodies and their souls – making them feel well, without diets.

13

Popular Diets and Nutrition Myths

At The Rooted Project, our main focus is helping people sort through nutri-nonsense. We do this because we feel strongly that people can't be empowered to make good decisions about their diet or health when they are basing their decisions on half-truths and misinformation. We spend a lot of time unpicking false claims and helping people to understand and weigh up the 'risks versus benefits' of different dietary approaches. This is so they can make decisions that are right for them, based on good information. There are so many fads, myths and trends out there, it would be impossible for us to squeeze in all the wacky things we've talked about over the years into the pages of this one book! What we can do (and have done) is put together a small collection of some of the more popular myths, fads and trends in nutrition, as it stands today. Here's your handy quick reference guide for some of the more hardy nutrition diets, trends and myths we've come across.

The Alkaline Diet

Diet: This diet removes 'acid-forming foods' and replaces them with 'alkaline-forming foods'. It's based around the theory that disease stems from acidity in the body caused by food.

Made popular by: This diet was made popular in the UK when Victoria Beckham was reported as a fan back in 2013, alongside other celebrities including Elle Macpherson and Gwyneth Paltrow.[1] [2] However, its original popularity sprung from the work of Robert O'Young, who published several books on the topic including *The pH Miracle*, which has sold millions of copies worldwide. (Note: Robert O'Young was sentenced to jail time in 2017 for illegally treating people at his ranch without any medical or scientific training.[3])

Mechanism and claims: When you metabolise foods they produce waste. These remaining chemicals can be either acidic or alkaline and are often referred to as 'ash' (a bit like the ash left over from burning fire in a stove). The acid/alkaline theory of disease, which the alkaline diet is based around, claims that this acid/alkaline 'ash' can have a direct effect on your health; acidic ash being disease-causing and alkaline ash, health promoting. This suggested mechanism has been widely criticised for being flawed. Your body's inbuilt regulatory systems (lungs and kidneys) keep your blood pH very tightly controlled and it isn't possible to change this with diet. You can, however, change the pH of your urine, which is what often draws people into the diet. Despite this, it's been claimed that this way of eating can protect your bones from weakening as you age (osteoporosis), protect your heart, fix depression and even cure and protect you from cancer.

Evidence: There have been a number of reviews of the alkaline diet to assess whether current evidence supports the claims made. Currently there is no evidence to support claims that an alkaline diet is an effective treatment or useful for prevention for any of the above conditions.[4] [5] [6] [7] [8]

Potential benefits: Most of the foods suggested on the alkaline diet are fresh fruits and vegetables, and many foods on the 'avoid' list are things like sweets, cakes and biscuits, etc., so that people who undertake this diet can see an improvement to the quality of their diet.

Risks: The alkaline diet does recommend avoiding high-protein 'acid'-forming foods like meat, fish and lentils (amongst other nutritious foods), so there is a risk that if the diet is not well planned you might miss out on beneficial nutrients. However, most of the risk lies with the way this diet is used. If you are rejecting proven medical therapies in favour of the alkaline diet as a treatment for cancer, for example, this diet can be very risky.

Bottom line: Most of us could do with eating more fruit and vegetables (lots of which would be alkaline-forming), but you don't need to refer to complicated lists, monitor your urine or avoid nutritious foods to safeguard your health. Personally, we would avoid the fad and concentrate on improving the overall quality of your diet in ways we know to be beneficial (e.g. increasing your fruit and veg consumption and making sure your alcohol and free-sugar intake is within recommended limits), rather than worrying about whether a food produces an acid or an alkaline 'ash' waste product.

Myth busting: detox diets

Detoxing is one of the cornerstones of wellness, claiming to help our bodies efficiently rid themselves of unwanted (and unnamed) toxins and they come in all different forms, from juice diets and supplements to detox teas and enema cleanses.

The need to detox seems to be born out of our obsession with purity and the guilt we feel for living a fast-paced, sometimes hedonistic lifestyle that makes us feel tired and drained. The idea that living at 100 miles an hour, drinking booze, smoking cigarettes and missing out on sleep can all be undone with a weekend ritual and cleanse is very appealing. The detox narrative plays on this and promotes the idea that our environments or lifestyles are 'toxic' and that we need to help cleanse ourselves to be healthy – and that our bodies need a helping hand to make this happen. Usually they involve a specific (and most of the time expensive) ritual or product we need to use, and in some cases a food we need to eat to 'speed up' the process. It's appealing as it's a quick fix (rather than the more time-consuming process of lifestyle changes, drink more water, eat more vegetables, get more sleep, etc).

There's no suggestion that you can't support your body by eating well and exercising, but your body has very sophisticated mechanisms for detoxing itself (your liver, kidneys, gut, skin and lungs all playing an important role). And although some animal studies have shown that a few foods might help support our bodies' natural detoxification pathways, there are currently no rigorous human trials that support the idea of an effective detox diet or any products that are known to make your body's natural detoxifying pathways any more efficient.

Carnivore

Diet: Meat only.

Made popular by: Mikhaila Peterson and her dad (clinical psychologist) Jordan Peterson. Another prominent advocate is Shawn Baker, a former orthopaedic surgeon.[9] [10]

Mechanism and claims: This diet has shot into the public domain after Mikhaila Peterson put her dad, a prominent psychologist (with somewhat controversial views) on the programme. She claims that the diet has cured her from severe arthritis, chronic fatigue, depression and many other symptoms she was previously experiencing.

Evidence: Although anecdotally there are people who claim this diet has worked wonders for them, there have been no observational studies or randomised controlled trials following people on a carnivore diet. Currently evidence is lacking to support the above claims or any health benefits for this diet.

Potential benefits: Unknown. It's possible a restrictive diet like this might provide relief via cutting out foods that someone is intolerant or allergic to, but this is quite a drastic and non-methodological way to eliminate potentially problematic foods.

Risks: This diet lacks variety, so the main risks are nutritional deficiencies, especially vitamin C. The lack of fibre in this diet also may have a knock-on effect on gut health (and you will probably get constipated or maybe not poo at all!).

Bottom line: This is a very extreme and restrictive diet with very little evidence to support its use.

Myth busting: turmeric tonics

Putting turmeric into drinks and tonics is currently a big thing in the wellness industry. It's claimed that its anti-inflammatory effects promote healthy brain ageing *and* decrease your risk of chronic health conditions like diabetes. It's also a popular alternative therapy for preventing and curing cancer.

But what do we really know? The part of turmeric thought to possess these beneficial properties is a compound called curcumin. Turmeric only contains teeny amounts of curcumin (max 5 per cent, but often as low as 2–3 per cent) which is very poorly absorbed from the spice. There are some compounds like piperidine (found in black pepper) that can significantly enhance the absorption of curcumin from turmeric, but even so, you're likely to need to eat a ton of the spice to get any beneficial effects (if there are any). That said, studies in test tubes have shown that turmeric has some potential as an anti-inflammatory/anti-cancer agent, but so far we have very few human experiments and most studies in people have found that they don't get a high enough dose from turmeric for it to have a medicinal effect.

This means that, as it stands, there's no good evidence to back up any of the health claims made about turmeric, but regularly using it in curries, drinking it in a tonic or having a turmeric latte may have a beneficial effect on your health over the long term (who knows?). However, its small potential as a healthy component of your diet shouldn't be confused with a cure-all or a 'natural' and safe replacement for modern medical therapies that have been shown to work. And while that might sound obvious, it isn't always. Any unsubstantiated treatments

▶

taken to extremes can be dangerous: one woman has died after being given an intravenous infusion of turmeric by her naturopathic doctor in the US.

So these trends might be harmless for many, but sometimes act as a 'gateway' to more insidious pseudoscientific nonsense. The fact that something is natural isn't a guarantee that it's safe or more effective than conventional medical therapies. Maybe curcumin will be used along with conventional cancer treatment one day, but at the moment It's way too early to tell.[11]

Intermittent Fasting

Diet: An eating pattern that alternates between periods of fasting and eating. Different variations all involve dividing the day or week into fasting and eating periods.

Made popular by: Ancient hunter-gatherers who at times would go through periods of fasting when food was scarce. A version of the diet, called the 5:2, became popular in 2012 after the BBC2 *Horizon* documentary, *Eat, Fast and Live Longer.*

Mechanism and claims: The premise is, when we intermittently fast, our body slows down into repair mode and there are beneficial changes in our body at a cellular level. These include an increase in insulin sensitivity and improvement in cellular repair. The idea is that this can help people lose weight, reduce the progression towards age-related diseases (such as cancer) and even improve longevity.

Evidence: Much of the research is in its early stages and many of the studies are short or have been carried out in animals. The 'CALERIE' study is currently underway in America, which is the first major human, randomised, controlled trial looking at the proposed long-term benefits of fasting, such as longer lifespan and decreased rates of cancer.[12] We know this happens in rats and several other mammals, but we can't directly translate this to humans without the proper trials.

Potential benefits: Some people find this way of eating extremely practical as it fits into their lifestyle better than the generic: breakfast/lunch/dinner framework.

Risks: Due to the calorie-restrictive nature of this way of eating, it might not be suitable for anyone with a history of eating disorders, trying to get pregnant, currently pregnant or breastfeeding.

Bottom line: IF may have promising health benefits such as protection against disease. That is if you like the idea of IF as a lifestyle choice and feel that it is something you can maintain in the long term.

Myth busting: plant lectins – are grains toxic for the gut?

Grains get a bad rap, with many people claiming that they are toxic and can cause damage to our gut lining, in turn causing 'leaky gut' (see page 175). One of the ways people suggest this happens is through lectins. Lectins are a type of indigestible

▶

protein found in grains and other foods, such as legumes, vegetables and even eggs, which can reduce absorption of carbohydrates. As we're unable to digest these proteins, they travel through our digestive system unchanged and in extremely large amounts, and it's thought that they could be damaging to the gut wall.

However, we don't eat lectins in isolation or in large enough amounts for them to be a problem. Uncooked grains and legumes have high amounts, but as long as you're cooking and preparing your food properly, they aren't something you need to worry about. Although it's common for people to focus on constituents of foods in order to label them good or bad, few foods are perfect. Grains do contain lectins, but they also contain gut-loving fibre and antioxidants, so the benefits far outweigh the risks. Diet patterns which are high in whole grains, like the Mediterranean diet, have been linked with healthy and long lives, so toxic grains is not something to worry about.

Keto

Diet: Very low-carb diet. There are various versions, but all usually require people to consume less than 20 grams of carbohydrates per day, replacing the carbs removed from the diet with fat.

Made popular by: This is a medical diet, often transiently prescribed for children with an epilepsy condition that doesn't respond to medication. More recently it's become a popular diet in the fitness industry for fat loss and as a potential treatment for people with type 2 diabetes.

Mechanism and claims: Reducing your carbohydrate intake to very low levels puts your body into ketosis: a metabolic state where you burn fat as your main source of fuel. The exact reason why this is helpful for people with epilepsy is poorly understood. However, proponents of this diet claim the subsequent reductions in insulin have health benefits, including management of type 2 diabetes and better metabolic health.

Evidence: A ketogenic diet can reduce seizures in children with epilepsy. A recent, very well-conducted, randomised controlled trial also showed that it may be an effective way for some people to manage type 2 diabetes. However, this diet is exceptionally hard to follow and even in study situations with lots of support, people find it extremely difficult to stick to.

Potential benefits: Can be used to manage epilepsy in children. It may be a useful tool for some people who have type 2 diabetes.[13]

Risks: There are many risks with this diet. Notable ones include low blood sugar, metabolic derangement, vitamin and mineral deficiency, stunted growth (in children), heart abnormalities and gut problems, like constipation. The health effects of following this diet in the long-term are also unknown.

Bottom line: This diet is extremely restrictive and hard to stick to. For some people with medical conditions it may be worth the difficulties and risks, but we strongly advise people not to follow a diet like this without medical supervision.

Myth busting: maca powder

Strange herbs and powders feature a lot in wellness regimes. Think skincare supplements, superfood powders and the modern-day alchemy found in brands like Moon Juice, which promise to tackle everything from improved sexual energy to boosting your brain power. Often these food supplements have fancy or exotic-sounding names, such as He Shou Wu or Reishi, making them seem mysterious and even exclusive. It's remarkably easy for self-styled influencers and health gurus to tap into this appeal and share anecdotes about why people in faraway lands take or use something, without having to provide any real evidence for its effects. In many ways this is harmless, as experimenting with food trends is fun! However, these strange herbs and powders are often very expensive and the claims around them can be wildly exaggerated. A really popular example of this right now is maca powder. Maca (or more specifically, maca root) is a plant native to Peru that has been used as a food and medicine by people in the Peruvian Andes for 1000–2000 years. More recently, its popularity as a herbal medicine has exploded, especially in China, where they have started cultivating this product to keep up with demand. It's claimed to fight fatigue and improve vigour, fertility, libido and memory. Some of the original, indigenous uses for maca have been stretched to breaking point to fit the booming demand for functional foods (foods that deliver a specific, health-giving nutrient) and herbal supplements.[14] It's not entirely clear how maca works; a few suggested mechanisms have been put forward, the most popular being that it contains large amounts of plant compounds that could be beneficial for your health, and,

▶

in particular, it's been discovered that they contain a group of compounds called 'macamides' (which is fun to say), which are unique to maca root. However, a recent review concluded that they were too small and had too many confounding factors to prove whether maca has any real effects. We also know very little about how much is safe to eat regularly. a recent review found that mass-cultivated maca had fewer macamides than the traditionally grown stuff and the amounts could vary widely. This means mass-produced maca could be widely different to the plants cultivated in the traditional way by villagers in the Peruvian Andes and that the purported benefits of Peruvian maca may not apply.

Juice Plus

Diet: Dried fruit and vegetable supplements, claimed to be the 'next best thing' to fruit and vegetables. These supplements are designed to be taken alongside your normal diet.

Made popular by: Multi-level marketing schemes. These tablets are often sold by people you know or who take them.

Mechanism and claims: Supplements are made from the dried juices of 30 fruits and vegetables. Although the company state on their website that these tables are not intended to replace fruits and vegetables, it's claimed they can improve your intake of nutrients, benefit your heart health, reduce stress and chronic inflammation, improve immune function, skin and even dental health.

Evidence: The company links to a lot of industry sponsored research on its website, which show that Juice Plus could increase your intake of nutrients.

Potential benefits: You may improve your intake of some micro-nutrients but there is no evidence these tablets are better than a regular multivitamin.

Risks: Gastro issues[15] and rashes[16] have been reported in science studies. It is also claimed that Juice Plus is aggressively promoted to cancer patients, due to its claimed antioxidant effects, but current evidence indicates that the potential risks of antioxidants outweigh the benefits when taken during cancer treatment.[17] They are also very expensive, retailing at around £37 a month.[18]

Bottom line: These tablets sound sexy, but powdered fruit and veg are not the same as their whole-food counterparts. There is also no evidence these can help cure cancer. Best to spare your wallet and stick to eating the real thing.

Myth busting: placenta pills

Now, sorry if you're squeamish, but this deep dive is about 'Placentophagia' – aka, consuming one's placenta!

The placenta is an organ that develops in the womb during pregnancy. This provides oxygen, hormones, antibodies and nutrients to the growing baby, plus it removes waste products from the baby's blood. Although mammals have

▶

historically eaten their placenta, this practice hasn't been common in the Western world until recent decades, where often educated, middle-class women are now choosing to eat their afterbirth.[19] The placenta is either eaten raw (e.g. within a fruit or veg smoothie), cooked (as a meat substitute), or most commonly sent off to be dehydrated, whizzed up into a powder and encapsulated (made into pills), costing about £200–300.

Placentophagy is rooted in the belief that ingesting the placenta provides benefits to the recovering postpartum mother. Advocates believe a host of benefits can be experienced, including increased energy, more rapid recovery, decreased incidence of baby blues and improved maternal bonding. Proponents believe these benefits are related to the placenta's excellent source of micronutrients – including dietary iron, which they believe helps restore women's iron levels that have been depleted during birth.

Some placenta encapsulation clinic websites we looked at cite results from human studies based on mothers self-reporting their experiences with placenta consumption (e.g. 'Taking the pills increased my energy levels and improved my breast milk supply'). This type of evidence is anecdotal, subject to bias and not considered to be high-quality under scientific standards. One study analysed the nutritional composition of 28 dehydrated placenta samples processed to be made into pills.[20] They found that the recommended daily allowance of the placenta pills would only provide a modest source of some micronutrients (24 per cent RDA for iron, 7.1 per cent RDA for selenium, 1.5 per cent RDA for zinc), so it was not the nutritional powerhouse it's often touted to be. This

▶

study also revealed that the samples contained levels of toxic elements (cyanide, arsenic, lead and mercury).

Although these levels were well below the toxic thresholds if taken within the recommended daily allowance of placenta pills (as they most commonly are), there is the risk that women consuming their placenta in more substantial quantities in other forms (e.g. raw within a smoothie) might risk overloading their body with toxic elements.

A small but rigorously designed, randomised, double-blind, placebo-controlled pilot study compared the iron levels of mothers consuming their own dehydrated placenta pills vs a placebo pill (dehydrated beef), whilst also meeting the RDA for dietary iron through their diet.[21] The findings indicated that the placenta pills did NOT significantly improve the mothers' iron levels and warrant a larger trial to confirm the results. The researchers concluded that this could be an important finding for mothers who are deficient in iron and whose only source of iron supplements is placenta pills, as these pills are likely to be inadequate and unable to rectify the deficiency. Another similarly designed pilot study found no robust differences in maternal mood, bonding or fatigue between the placenta or beef placebo groups.

One issue is that the process of encapsulating the placenta is not standardised or regulated (although measures are being made to do so), which means the treatment of one placenta may be different to another. This is a worrying health and safety concern – we're talking about handling human tissue here – and leaves scope for variation in the nutrient content of different capsules (despite reassurances from the practitioner in question).[22]

▶

Overall, although mammals have historically eaten their own placenta, it doesn't necessarily mean we should! Women who have taken part in the practice speak of the many benefits, despite lack of evidence. Placenta pills show no difference in effect on the maternal iron status of women post-birth than a beef placebo. They are also likely to be an insufficient source of iron for women who are iron-deficient following birth. More research is needed to see what happens to this group of women who rely on placenta pills as their sole iron supplement.

Despite its popularity, there is no robust scientific evidence yet that eating the placenta post-birth provides objectively demonstrable benefits for the mother beyond a placebo effect.

14

Exploring Evidence

Although the common view of science is that it's an ever-expanding body of knowledge and facts, the awkward truth is that science itself isn't about 'proof' or certainty or providing simple black-and-white answers, it's about limiting doubt. In fact, it's very rare to find absolute certainty in science, which is why researchers and scientists always seem to be adding caveats to statements or won't give a straight answer – because there isn't one.

So, given our aim is to empower you to make informed choices, it'd be remiss of us if we didn't include a chapter showing you how to pick through nutrition information. Nutrition science is one of the most complex, fascinating and (in many ways) maddening sciences out there. Simply being aware of this can be a huge advantage, but we're going to go a little further and give you tools to sort fact from fiction when you're reading nutrition information in the real world.

Since the digital revolution launched us into an age of information, we've dramatically changed the way we work and learn. It started with the internet's slow and clunky introduction to our households in the 90s (screeching into action with that nostalgic dial-up tone) and since then, both the volume of information and speed at which we can access it has skyrocketed. We're exposed to massive amounts of information daily and can find out nearly anything we want to know at the click of a button. This has been transformative for the democratisation of information: we no longer need the approval of big publications or mass-media outlets to connect us to an audience. Everyone has a voice and absolutely anyone can put themselves out there and spread their message through their own YouTube channels, blogs and social media accounts.

Naturally, it's a double-edged sword and this unlimited access to unfiltered content isn't always positive. Information can be shaped, spun and curated to suit any agenda and even with the best will in the world, none of it can be truly without bias. In fact, it's precisely this incredible 'free for all' access that dilutes quality information with opinion and anecdotes, so ultimately, we lose any sense of the 'truth' amidst the swathes of conspiracies theories, unfounded beliefs and propaganda that fill up our news feeds.

To pick through it all, one of the most important skills we can develop is the ability to 'see' good information and filter out the bad. And that's no mean feat: nutrition is one of the most contentious sciences out there, the nuanced discussion of the issues (which we promise is out there!) is too often clouded by media misrepresentation and popular personal narratives.

Talking point: why we get sucked into nutrition nonsense

Nutrition myths masquerading as health or medical advice are everywhere, and despite us being the sentient and intelligent beings that we are, with unlimited access to good, solid evidence-based info online, it's still so easy to fall into the trap of believing in nutrition nonsense. Let's look at some of the reasons why nutri-nonsense is so appealing to us.

Appeal to nature: The idea that something is natural so it must be good is a common one in nutrition. It appeals to the comforting belief that the world provides for us. Saying something is 'natural' sounds like it's gentle, wholesome and unprocessed. It's a term tapped into by people in advertising and product production, because we automatically associate it with 'better for us'. However, natural is an ambiguous term – it isn't a guarantee that something is safe or effective. Cyanide is 'natural', for example.

Appeal to authority: This is one of the easiest ones to spot. If someone is asking you to believe information based on their title or the qualifications they hold, be wary. 'Trust me I'm a doctor/nutritionist/scientist' isn't good reasoning. If an opinion is grounded in evidence, people should be able to tell you why they think what they think and, most importantly, how they came to that conclusion.

Appeal to ancient wisdom: This narrative suggests that if a practice is old it must be beneficial, otherwise why are we still doing it? Or if a piece of knowledge has survived the test of

▶

time, it must be true. These ancient wisdoms are often simple rules or practices that are easily applied to our everyday lives, making them really appealing in a sea of confusing messages. However, just because something is old doesn't make it true or helpful!

Appeal to novelty: Strange herbs and powders, especially if they are old AND from far away can be really appealing and exciting. It's also easy for people to share anecdotes about why people in faraway lands take or use something, without having to provide any real evidence for its effects. Experimenting with food trends is fun! However, these foods are often very expensive and the claims around them can be wildly exaggerated.

A thread of science: Many nutrition myths are based around a little bit of science. This reference to the recognisable but complex can fool us into thinking that the claims being made are grounded in scientific reasoning. A good example of this is IV vitamin drips (the trendy practice of having your vitamins infused directly into your bloodstream). It sounds kind of sensible, right? Vitamins are good for you, we need them, they are 'natural', so this is probably harmless and having more should be better. Also, they are given in clinics by doctors and nurses, so they seem sciencey and must be legit? But that's sadly not the case – unless your bowel isn't working, there's really no need to risk infection and take your vitamins IV.

The Dunning-Kruger Effect:

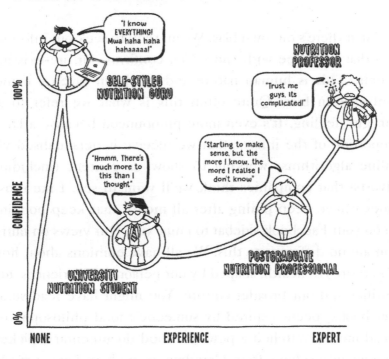

The more you know, the more you realise how much you don't know. The Dunning-Kruger Effect speaks to the phenomenon where people with the least experience and knowledge talk with confidence and authority, because they have no idea how limited their knowledge actually is. At the same time, someone with years of experience can appear non-committal or as though they doubt their position, due to the caveating statements and sharing their uncertainty. If someone is handing you a silver bullet and offering you a simple fix, be wary: our desire for certainty can blind us to the fact that the gurus are just confidently wrong.

Then there's our own bias. We all tend to seek out information that we agree with and which confirms our pre-existing beliefs. This is human nature and has been given a name: confirmation bias. Quite often this is what we refer to as our 'gut' feeling. It's even more pronounced because a large proportion of the information we receive is personalised via online algorithms, working to show us content (including adverts) that companies think we'll want to see. Like those shoes you've been pining after all month that keep popping up on your Facebook sidebar to taunt you. Our views on nutrition are no different to this. We all have opinions about how food relates to health, shaped by our personal experiences, our families and our broader culture. You might have read some diet books, been inspired by someone's food philosophy on social media, watched a powerful food documentary, picked up ancient wisdoms from Grandma, or perhaps have a medical condition that requires you to follow a special diet. These unconscious preferences or beliefs (biases) are everywhere and help to build your own food-health world, so it can be

HIERARCHY
OF
EVIDENCE

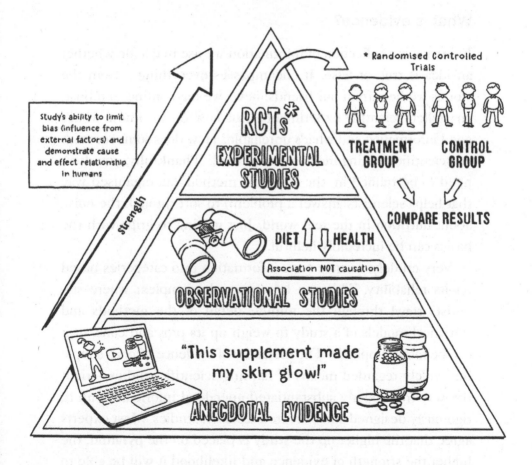

* Randomised Controlled Trials

Study's ability to limit bias (influence from external factors) and demonstrate cause and effect relationship in humans

strength

RCTs*
EXPERIMENTAL STUDIES

TREATMENT GROUP

CONTROL GROUP

COMPARE RESULTS

DIET ⬆⬇ HEALTH

Association NOT causation

OBSERVATIONAL STUDIES

"This supplement made my skin glow!"

ANECDOTAL EVIDENCE

a challenge to see things from another perspective. Being
able to take a step back and recognise bias is key if you're
hoping to avoid nutri-nonsense. This is one of the benefits
of the scientific method – it's self-critical and (over time)
self-correcting. It uses specific systematic methods, with
the hope of minimising bias, so we can be sure if our views
are grounded in fact and not a product of our own skewed
perceptions.

So let's start at the beginning.

What is evidence?

Evidence is a collection of information we use to decide whether
an idea is true or false. It encompasses everything – from the
stories we hear from our friends, news we read online to robust,
controlled scientific experiments. But how do we know what's
good information and what's unreliable? How does someone with
no scientific training make sense of it all? Thankfully, you don't
need to be trained in 'the scientific method' (an organised way
that helps scientists answer a problem) to sort through the noise
about nutrition in the real world. Just getting to grips with the
basics can be incredibly helpful.

Very crudely, science sorts information into categories based
on its reliability. This can be extremely complex; where scientists trawl through the minute detail of the methods and
statistical models of a study to weigh up its pros and cons, or it
can be more simplistic. The hierarchy of evidence offers a simple
but widely regarded means of ranking scientific studies – right
the way from poorly substantiated anecdotal information up to
rigorously designed and executed research studies. Most experts
agree that the higher up the study is placed on the pyramid, the
higher the strength of evidence and likelihood it will be able to

establish cause and effect relationships (e.g. this food has this effect on the body).

Type of evidence	What does this mean?	Strengths	Weaknesses
Systematic reviews	Multiple studies are combined to create a 'mega study', providing an unbiased overview of the best available evidence.		
Clinical trials	Researchers ask people to adopt a new behaviour (such as eating a special diet or taking a supplement) and see if it affects their health.	Can compare the intervention with a control or placebo. In randomised controlled trials, one group typically receives the intervention and the other does not. Conditions can be controlled. Can prove cause and effect. Can apply study findings to a group of people.	Study results can't always be applied to the whole population. Some diets can't be tested due to ethical reasons (e.g. trialling a new supplement on pregnant women).
Observational studies	Scientists track the habits of a large group of people going about their normal life to see if any associations can be found between a food/supplement and health outcome.	Can raise interesting questions to follow up in human clinical trials.	Variables can't be controlled for that might affect health outcomes, e.g. some study participants might have regularly drunk orange juice (high in vitamin C) which could skew the results. Only associations can be drawn upon. Correlation does not equal causation.
Animal studies	Scientists feed animals a particular diet or supplement and measure its effect on their health.		Humans are not mice! We can't apply these findings to human beings.

Type of evidence	What does this mean?	Strengths	Weaknesses
In vitro studies	Researchers explore the effect that a food or nutrient has on a tissue, cell or molecule.		Humans are not skin cells, we're a complex collection of cells, tissues and organs, living free in the world! We can't apply these findings to human beings.
Anecdote or expert opinion	Evidence in the form of stories that people tell to recount their experiences or the opinion from an expert in nutrition.		

These different methods all have their strengths and weaknesses, but they can be used to build a picture, so we can better see what is going on. Observational studies track the habits of large groups of people to see if any trends can be found, lab and animal studies can be used to explain *how* these patterns may occur by establishing the underlying biological mechanism, and experimental studies (or randomised controlled trials) can be designed to compare one group against another in a way that means we can truly see if an effect occurs or whether it's all an illusion.

We just want to clarify that this hierarchy is only a general guideline, not an absolute rule. To the trained eye, there are certainly cases where a nutrition study lower down the pyramid could provide more value and insight than a study with a more robust design. The research methods within this hierarchy can be read about in more detail in the appendix but for those not interested in the nitty gritty, the simple rule you have to remember is this central point: in nutrition, no single study alone can tell us much of anything. You have you look at the entire body of research, not just one or two papers.

In nutrition, we need all of them. And there's a reason for this.

Despite the clear advantages of conducting a randomised controlled trial, only a small fraction of human nutrition studies are designed in this way. Instead, we have decades of observational studies that can show us trends and patterns but can't be used to prove 'cause and effect', like the neat experimental trials used in the medical world. So why aren't there more randomised controlled trials in nutrition science?

Nutrition is a 'messy science' which is deeply difficult to study. When scientists have a theory about a food or a diet, they're ultimately interested in what happens to our health over the long term, not what happens over the course of a few weeks, months or (even years!). But you can't confine a study participant for decades, monitoring every last morsel of food they put into their mouth and controlling each minute of their life. Even if you could, the results you generated would be meaningless in the real world, where people behave like the unpredictable, erratic beings that we are. Running meaningful, large, long-term RCTs to definitively answer those big, important questions (such as which diets cause cancer), is likely to be expensive and extremely impractical. For example, to collect truly definitive data, scientists may arguably need to randomise thousands of children at birth, force them to follow either a diet full of fruits and veggies or cola and chocolate and monitor their whole lives to note who developed cancer, depression, died young or aged well. But obviously that's a bit too much of a dystopian nightmare. Even on a voluntary basis, can you imagine being asked to follow a set diet for decades? And how would you feel if the diet you were required to follow was extremely restrictive, or wasn't making you feel so good? These trials can only help us answer short-term questions, such as the effect of a food on bowel movement or blood cholesterol levels. This means that most studies in nutrition are observational, so they can't show us cause and effect. This doesn't make them useless; it does mean that they require careful interpretation and a mix of all different study types to help us build up a better picture of what effects different diets and foods have.

What's evidence-based practice?

An evidence-based practice is more than just reading and understanding the science; it involves the use of scientific literature to inform recommendations for public policy or any other form of communication, or to help people make a decision that is right for their unique circumstances. In addition to this, true evidence-based practitioners know the limitations of their own knowledge, and when and where to seek help and support. This practice, as you can imagine, is a skill which takes time, effort and experience to develop. But right now, claiming to be 'evidence-based' has become a bit of a trend. Sadly (but predictably) this rise in popularity means that the term has also been hijacked by people keen to boost their credibility, even if they aren't exactly adhering to its principles. There are literally hundreds and thousands of people (including us!) claiming to use an evidence-based approach, many of whom have totally opposing views on what's 'fact' or 'backed by science'. You'll see people promoting single eating styles as 'the best' or posting and quoting single studies to support their viewpoint, or 'prove' that they are correct.

So what should we do?

The easiest way to decipher if someone's view is grounded in evidence is to ask them *how* they came to their views. Any sound, evidence-based practitioner should be able to share their method with you. But there are other tell-tales signs that people might be trying to pull the wool over your eyes that you can look out for, too.

Spotting nutrition quacks

Choosing where to get our info from can be just as much of a minefield as knowing what it really means. One of the first things we often look for when seeking somebody's expertise is their authority, usually in the form of credentials and titles. However, authority can be misleading. Dr Gillian McKeith PhD, a noughties', self-styled nutritionist and prime-time TV celebrity, oozed authority with her white coat, jazzy science lingo and obsession with poo-themed laboratory tests. Her credibility was also enforced through her strong media presence; she was extremely popular in the worlds of television and publishing, gracing our screens and publishing books that climbed to the top of the bestseller charts. The public only later discovered that Gillian's PhD was obtained via distance learning from an unaccredited holistic nutrition college. The Advertising Standards Authority promptly ruled that any adverts linked to McKeith using the title Dr were misleading and could not run. She was not a medical doctor nor a qualified nutritionist, but she fell into a clinical stereotype and sounded like she knew what she was talking about, so we believed her.

Although we no longer have Gillian, there is always the opportunity to take our nutrition advice from other non-credible sources. New wellness experts, health coaches and eating disorder specialists (without a qualification to their name) are popping up all over the place. More difficult to spot, however, are those like McKeith, but with actual legitimate qualifications. Doctors interested in 'lifestyle medicine' but with little experience in the complexities of critiquing and applying nutrition science to public health and clinical practice are inadvertently driving confusion by pushing for single, over-simple solutions to poor health, such as low-carb diets for all. This appeal to authority and credentials and accolades over evidence is rife in nutrition, and coupled with the hype of the headlines this leads to a confusing mass of mixed messages. So in striving to be objective, it's crucial to be aware of the prevalence of subtle manipulation in our media-heavy lives. Open-minded scepticism is the order of the day when it comes to claims about health and nutrition. In other words, we advocate taking the majority of information thrown our way on that front with a large pinch of (pink Himalayan) salt.

Talking point: nutrition myths in wellness culture

Anthony Warner (The Angry Chef)

I spent quite a lot of time researching the dark side of wellness and diet culture, and there are some common themes. Messages generally tap into some of our innate desires. One of the most important is our desire for simplicity. We are strongly drawn to simple messages, rules that make the complexity of life easier to navigate. Sadly, often this is something that real nutrition science struggles to provide, because it is such an uncertain and nuanced science with a great deal of complexity. People with qualifications, experience and integrity will rarely give you a simple dietary rule to live by, and advice is usually along the lines of 'eat a balanced diet, not too much or too little, plenty of variety, lots of fruits and vegetables, a bit of oily fish'. This still leaves us with lots of complex decisions to make for ourselves and doesn't really give us a simple rule about what the 'best' diet is. When some shiny, but completely unqualified, diet guru comes along and gives you definitive rules about what you should be eating, those messages have

▶

instinctive appeal. They will say things like 'gluten is the devil, sugar is toxic, kale cures disease and green juices make you live longer', despite there being no good evidence that this is the case. They give us simple shortcuts and make navigating the world easier, so often we are inclined to believe them more than the subtle, nuanced (and factual) messages that evidence-based science provides.

Here's our list of red flags to look out for when spotting nutri-nonsense

- Appeals to their title/authority as a reason to trust them, not evidence and reasoning.
- Uses anecdotes as sole source of evidence.
- Deals in absolutes or single approaches, without reference to the uncertainties and nuance of nutrition science, e.g. one best diet for everyone.
- Uses sensationalist and fear-promoting language like 'toxic' or poisonous.
- Promotes quick fixes and miracle cures.
- References conspiracies, e.g. 'Things your doctor doesn't want you to know.'
- Promotes complementary treatments as a sole alternative to medical care.
- Focuses on natural as superior to synthetic.
- Sells supplements or detox programmes.
- Focuses on nutrition as the sole cause and cure of diseases.
- Appeals to ancient wisdom, or the idea that natural is always best.

Evaluating nutrition stories in the news

Learning to read and evaluate scientific studies (particularly in nutrition) is a skill that takes a long time to develop. Despite the easy access now to research abstracts on sites like 'PubMed', simply sticking a subject into Google and reading a few research summaries does not make you a scientist. However, you don't need to become an expert or spend years learning to read scientific research to be able to successfully navigate the media spin. There are a few things that you can look out for when reading stories about nutrition and health that can be helpful when making a judgment on how accurate and applicable the information in front of you is to your life.

Publication quality

Are you reading a press release? A carefully curated PR communication sitting pretty as an apparent information piece? Is it in the tabloids?! You get the picture. Considering the reliability and quality of a publication, including their inherent ideologies and bias, is useful for putting stories into context.

Peer review

The first thing to note is whether the article you are reading is discussing research that has been 'peer reviewed'. Once a study is complete and the researchers want to share their work, they approach journals for publication, but this is not an easy process (and for good reason). To reliably evaluate the quality of the research in a scientific paper, the study's methodology is analysed by a board of scientists who rigorously evaluate the work to confirm that it meets the standards we outlined earlier. However, sometimes the press will report findings of studies which have yet to go through this process, or opinion pieces that aren't subject to peer review as if they are on equal footing to actual research which has been through this process.

Study funding

Science is not perfect, and since research is expensive, it can often be funded by industries that have a vested interest in the outcome. In fact, multiple studies have shown us that research sponsored by industry is much more likely to produce positive results than studies funded by other sources (e.g. government bodies). If a study has been funded by industry, it doesn't completely invalidate the results, but it's worth considering that the results may be overblown or a little misleading.

Relative or absolute risk?

Statistics in health stories in the news are selected to sound as dramatic as possible: *Eating processed meat increases your risk of breast cancer by 21 per cent.* What these numbers are describing is 'relative risk': a number that tells us how much more or less likely one group is to develop a disease or condition than another. While relative risk can help us understand that a behaviour may increase our risk of poor health, it tells us nothing about how big or small our individual risk is. This means that the percentages can sound big and scary, but the increase in our actual, individual risk depends on what our risk was in the first place. This can be influenced by our age, genetics, social and financial status and also our lifestyle (to name just a few). So the real question is: '21 per cent of what?' If your risk of breast cancer is relatively small, say one in 1000, a 21 per cent increase raises this to 1.2 in 1000, which is essentially the same, as we don't tend to divide people into fractions. Even a 100 per cent increase is a relatively small, at two in 1000. If your individual risk is larger, perhaps you are a postmenopausal woman and breast cancer runs in your family, it may mean that these studies (and the risk increase) may be more relevant to you and a consideration for your lifestyle.

You are not a mouse

The final key concept is quite a straightforward one. You are not a mouse. Or a rat. Or a monkey. Animal studies are often used to help us predict the effects of something in a whole living body, as it's so much more complex than testing individual cells in a test tube. But despite being useful for highlighting scientific theories that might be worth exploring further, the fact is that animal studies don't reliably predict the effects of diets or treatments in humans and we can't apply the data from animal studies to people. It certainly can't be used to inform public health advice, so just keep an eye out for any lifestyle recommendations founded on the caffeine response of Barry the Mouse.

Putting this knowledge into practice

A unicorn's guide to spotting bad science in the press

Don't take an article's word for it.

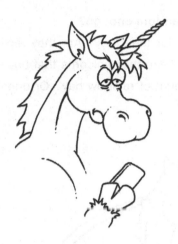

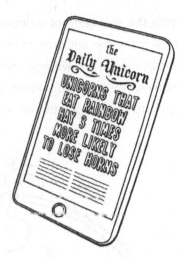

Go to the study source.
Was the study published in a peer-reviewed journal? And was the study done in a group relevant to you – e.g. was it on old unicorns, female unicorns, or maybe even horses?

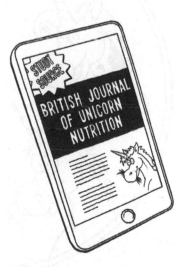

Did the study ask enough unicorns (if it wasn't done in a test tube)?

The number of unicorns included in the study will affect how likely it is that the results are true and not down to chance (more unicorns = better).

Was the selection of unicorns random enough?

How were the unicorns recruited for the study? Are they representative of an average unicorn? Are they unicorns that have been exposed to an unusual amount of rainbow hay? Or ones that are more prone to horn loss?

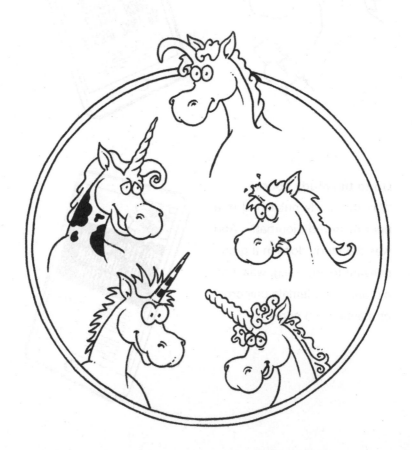

Was there a control group to check the rainbow hay was really to blame?

Ideally the number of horns lost in a group of unicorns eating rainbow hay should be compared to those eating regular yellow hay to see if there is a difference between the two groups. This will tell you if this is a regular amount of horns that can be expected to be lost, or if rainbow hay increases the risk of horn loss.

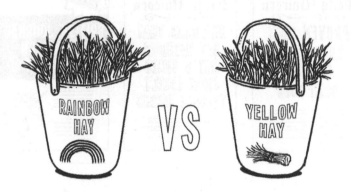

Who funded the study?

Check to see if this study was funded by any other industry organisations that might want to sway the results of the study.

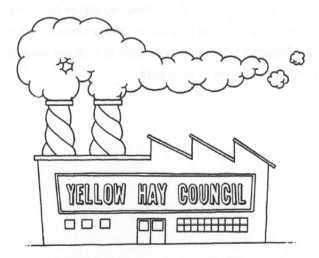

How was the story reported?

Watch out for sensationalist newspaper headlines. Especially those containing words 'proves' or 'causes'. Science is often not clear cut and journalists should use caveats to report findings.

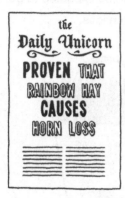 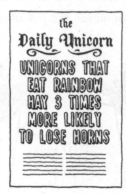 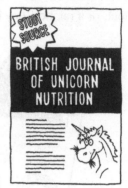

Understand how the risk of harm (e.g. unicorn horn loss) has been presented. It might not be as scary as the article implies.

Check out the 'absolute risk'. This will tell you more about your actual risk of horn loss. E.g. if 'rainbow hay triples horn loss risk' from one in 2000 unicorns to three in 2000 unicorns your absolute risk of losing a horn goes from 0.05 to 0.15 per cent. So it's still a pretty low chance of horn loss.

Closing Thoughts

This book is packed with information about nutrition – we hope you found it helpful and that at least some of it will stick with you while you navigate all the crazy messages about food that you come across in your daily life. We also hope you picked up on a few of the common themes that cropped up throughout.

The first is that while the things you eat can have an impact on your health, food is so much more than a collection of nutrients or a vehicle through which to achieve 'healthy'. Food is social and joyful and emotional. It's your Grandma's Lancashire hotpot with your family, cake on your birthday, the Thai meal you ate with your partner on your first date. It's something that's great to pay a little attention to, but it's also something that should bring you pleasure and joy.

The second is that nutrition science is a complicated process – the young hot mess of the science world that is still finding its feet. There is so much we don't yet know, and while this makes it a super exciting area to study, it can (and has) resulted in lots of confusing and conflicting messages. We hope that reading this book has given you a grounding in the basics and the knowledge to navigate this environment a little better.

Finally (and probably most importantly), we want to stress that there's really no such thing as a perfect diet. Health isn't something you find in a formulaic way to eat, or at the bottom of a perfectly presented smoothie bowl. There are many roads to good health. Your dietary needs and what's 'best' for you will also change, not because dietary advice changes or because you suddenly decided to give up meat, but because life is busy. Sometimes the best thing for your health will be four weeks straight of ready meals, because you're studying for exams and don't have time to cook. You might be a new mum or find yourself living in a poky flat with only a microwave to work with. You might 'ahem' find yourself eating a custard tart for dinner and sipping coffee at 11pm in order to meet a deadline for your book edits ... You get the picture.

Overall, we really hope the tools in this book give you the assurance to navigate eating with confidence and allow you to eat freely, without guilt or confusion. Screw the fads, the silver bullets and the quick-fix diets. We encourage you to find what works for you – to eat your veggies, move your body in a way that brings you joy, include foods you love in your diet and, most of all, to have fun! You've got this.

Appendix

Micronutrients: requirements and doses

Nutrient	Food sources	How much do I need? (per day)*	What if I don't get enough?	Can I have too much?*
Vitamin C	Oranges Lemons Kiwi Blackcurrants Mangoes Papaya Guava Peppers Broccoli Brussels sprouts Sweet potatoes Liver and kidney	<1 year old: 25mg 1–10 years: 30mg 11–14 years: 35mg >15 years: 40mg Pregnancy 1st & 2nd trimester: 40mg 3rd trimester: 50mg Breastfeeding: 70mg Regular smokers: 80mg	May cause thickening of the skin and poor wound healing. Can lead to a condition called 'scurvy', which causes weakness, tiredness, irritability, sore limbs, bleeding gums, bleeding skin, skin discoloration and bruises.	We pee out most of the extra vitamin C that our body does not need, which reduces the risk of harm from having too much. However, a very high intake from supplements can cause diarrhoea and increase the risk of kidney stones. The UK Department of Health advises that up to 1000mg of vitamin C supplements per day is unlikely to cause any harm.
B vitamins	Whole-grain products (like bread, pasta, rice, cereals) Meats Eggs Dairy products Yeast products (like Marmite and nutritional yeast) Some fortified breakfast cereals	Adults need: Thiamine (B1) Women: 1mg Men: 1.4mg Riboflavin (B2) Women: 1.1mg Men: 1.3mg Niacin acid (B3): Women: 13mg Men: 17mg Pantothenic acid (B5): roughly 3–7mg Pyridoxine (B6): Women: 1.2mg Men: 1.4mg Biotin (B7): 10– 200µg	This could cause you to feel tired, weak, irritable or low in mood. May also cause diarrhoea, skin problems, or mouth and tongue sores. Severely low levels can lead to medical issues with our heart and nervous system (including our brain).	It is advised to get our B vitamins from our food, but if you use supplements these are the estimated safe amounts per day: Thiamine (B1): <100mg Riboflavin: <40mg Nicotinamide (a form of B3): <500mg Pantothenic acid (B5): 200mg Pyridoxine (B6) <10mg Biotin (B7): <900µg Large doses of pantothenic acid (B5) may cause diarrhoea.

Nutrient	Food sources	How much do I need? (per day)*	What if I don't get enough?	Can I have too much?*
Folic acid (or folate)	Folic acid supplements Folic acid found in food is called folate, this is found in most fruit and vegetables (especially green leafy vegetables), beans, peas, fortified breakfast cereals, whole grains, nuts, dairy products, eggs and meat	<1 year: 50µg 1–3 years: 70µg 4–6 years: 100µg 7–10 years: 150µg >11 years: 200µg Pregnancy: 300µg Planning a pregnancy and until the 12th week of pregnancy: 400µg Pregnant women with an increased risk of neural tube defects (NTDs) for the baby: 5000µg	May cause diarrhoea. Can increase the risk of infertility. Can cause a type of anaemia where your body creates unusually large blood cells that can't carry oxygen around your body properly (megaloblastic anaemia). When planning a pregnancy, and up to the 12th week of pregnancy, a low intake can increase the risk of neural tube defects (like spina bifida) in the baby.	There is a low risk that a high intake of folate causes harm. Folic acid supplements can hide the symptoms of vitamin B12 deficiency. Remember that folic acid supplements are essential in early pregnancy to reduce the risk of NTDs.
Vitamin B12	Meat Fish Eggs Dairy products Yeast products (like Marmite and nutritional yeast) Breakfast cereals fortified with vitamin B12	0–6 months: 0.3µg 7–12 months: 0.4µg 1–3 years: 0.5µg 4–6 years: 0.8µg 7–10 years: 1.0µg 11–14 years: 1.2µg >15 years: 1.5µg 19–50 years: 1.5µg Breastfeeding: 2µg	May mean that your body cannot properly use the energy from your food. Can cause the same type of anaemia that is caused by not having enough folate (megaloblastic anaemia). May cause harm to the nervous system, which can lead to limb weakness, numbness or tingling, and in some cases problems with memory and brain function.	There is a low risk of harm related to high intakes of vitamin B12. The UK Department of Health advises that up to 2000µg of B12 supplements per day is unlikely to cause any harm.

Nutrient	Food sources	How much do I need? (per day)*	What if I don't get enough?	Can I have too much?*
Vitamin A (retinol and beta-carotene)	Retinol: liver, kidney, oily fish, fish liver oils, eggs, fortified spreads and dairy products Beta-carotene: carrots, red peppers, tomatoes, broccoli and spinach	<1 years: 350µg (or retinol equivalent) 1–3 years: 400µg 4–10 years: 500µg 11–14 years: 600µg >15 years: Women: 600µg Men: 700µg Pregnancy: 700µg Breastfeeding: 950µg	Can cause sight problems like night blindness and dry eyes. May also cause skin problems such as causing dead skin cells to block pores. Can increase the risk of infection. May reduce male fertility and cause problems in pregnancy.	Too much vitamin A can cause abdominal pain, vomiting, irritability, headaches, blurred vision, hair loss and damage to the skin, eyes, bones and liver. Too much vitamin A can harm an unborn baby, so it is very important that women who are pregnant or planning a pregnancy should not take supplements containing vitamin A (unless advised to do so by a doctor) and should avoid eating liver. The rest of the population is advised not to eat liver more than once per week.
Vitamin D	Cod liver oil Oily fish Dairy products Egg yolks Red meat Liver Fortified margarine Fortified breakfast cereals The best source of vitamin D is sunlight or vitamin D supplements	<1 year: 8.5-10µg >1 year: 10µg Pregnancy: 10µg Breastfeeding: 10µg	Can contribute to bone weakness problems like rickets and osteomalacia. May also increase the risk of illness and infection .	It is not possible to get too much vitamin D from the sun (but there is a risk of skin damage from UV rays). Too much vitamin D from supplements can damage the bones, kidneys and heart (but this is rare). The UK Department of Health advises that up to 100µg of vitamin D supplements for adults, 50µg for children 1–10 years old, and 25µg for infants <1 year old is unlikely to be harmful.

Nutrient	Food sources	How much do I need? (per day)*	What if I don't get enough?	Can I have too much?*
Vitamin E	Olive oil Rapeseed oil Corn oil Soya bean oil Sunflower oil Safflower oil Nuts Seeds Whole-grain products	Women: 3mg Men: 4mg Pregnancy: 3.8–6.2mg Breastfeeding: 3.8–6.2mg	May increase the risk of illness and infection. We also need enough vitamin E to keep our muscles, skin and eyes healthy.	Too much vitamin E can reduce the amount of vitamins A, D and K that we absorb cause weakness, headaches, muscle weakness, double vision and stomach pain. It is advised to get vitamin E from our diet instead of supplements, but having up to 540mg of vitamin E from supplements is unlikely to be harmful.
Vitamin K	Green leafy vegetables (like spinach, kale, broccoli and cabbage) Soya bean oil Walnut oil Olive oil Rapeseed oil Sesame oil Eggs Meat Dairy products Our gut bacteria also make vitamin K for our body to use	1µg per kg of body weight, e.g. if you weigh 70kg you would need about 70µg of vitamin K per day	Could cause poor blood clotting, poor wound healing or bile duct problems. Low levels of vitamin K are rare.	As the body stores leftover vitamin K, having too much could cause damage to our liver or brain. It is advised to get vitamin K from a balanced diet, but if you do take supplements, having up to 1mg of vitamin K is unlikely to cause harm. Vitamin K supplements are not advised if you take blood thinning medication (like warfarin).

Nutrient	Food sources	How much do I need? (per day)*	What if I don't get enough?	Can I have too much?*
Calcium	Dairy products (like milk, yoghurt and cheese) Fortified dairy alternatives (like soya or almond milk) Green leafy vegetables Beans Lentils Chickpeas Tofu Nuts Bread Tinned fish (with bones)	<1 year: 525mg 1–3 years: 350mg 4–6 years: 450mg 7–10 years: 550mg 11–18 years Girls: 800mg Bcys: 1000mg >18 years: 700mg Breastfeeding: 1250mg	Low intake in childhood can stunt growth. Can increase the risk of brittle bones and cause rickets in childhood, or osteoporosis in later life. Calcium is needed for blood clotting and to keep our teeth and muscles healthy.	Having more than 1500mg of calcium in one day could cause diarrhoea and stomach pains. But having less than 1500mg per day is unlikely to be harmful.
Iodine	Fish Shellfish Seaweed Dairy products Iodised salt	3 months: 50µg 4–12 months: 60µg 1–3 years: 70µg 4–6 years: 100µg 7–10 years: 110µg 11–14 years: 130µg > 15 years: 140µg	Low intakes may cause hypo-thyroidism, which in turn can cause swelling if the thyroid gland (goitre), tiredness, poor concentration, dry skin, weight gain and a reduced heart rate. This can also cause infertility and problems during pregnancy, including an increased risk of cretinism for the baby (stunted physical and mental development).	Taking too much iodine over a long period of time can cause harm to our thyroid gland (and increase the risk of hyperthyroidism). It is advised to get iodine from our food, but if you do use a supplement, having up to 500µg of iodine per day is unlikely to be harmful.

Nutrient	Food sources	How much do I need? (per day)*	What if I don't get enough?	Can I have too much?*
Iron	Liver Meat Poultry Fish Eggs Beans Nuts Dried fruit – such as apricots Whole grains Fortified breakfast cereals Yeast extract Green leafy vegetables (like kale, spinach and watercress)	0–3 months: 1.7mg 4–6 months: 4.3mg 7–12 months: 7.8mg 1–3 years: 6.9mg 4–6 years: 6.1mg 7–10 years: 8.7mg 11–18 years Girls: 14.8mg Boys: 11.3mg 19–50 years Women: 14.8mg Men: 8.7mg > 50 years: 8.7mg	Can cause anaemia, which means that blood cells which can't carry oxygen around your body properly. Signs of low iron include being pale, tired, insomnia, shortness of breath and heart palpitations.	Taking supplements with up to 17mg of iron per day is unlikely to be harmful (but it's important to continue taking a higher dose if advised to by your doctor. Having more than 20mg of iron can cause nausea, vomiting, constipation, stomach pain and reduced absorption of other nutrients (like zinc).

* This information is based on UK guidelines. µg = micrograms (i.e. one-thousandth of a milligram)

Label reading

This book has hopefully unpicked some of the most pressing concerns when it comes to eating well, but there is one more area we think warrants some airtime. Possibly the most prosaic demonstration of our relationship with food is the food label. These images and words on packets are there to protect us and can help us to make informed decisions when shopping, but they can be confusing – especially as these bottles and wrappers are the manufacturer's chance to push their sales pitch. What's fascinating is when looked at from a historical perspective, these labels on food reflect the politics and our judgements from that era: what we deem to be a risk, good or important for health.

Food laws have not always existed and, historically, manu-facturers could effectively get away with murder. It was during the Industrial Revolution, when people moved towards towns and cities, that the public started to become more dependent on packaged food. With this came 'food adulteration': the addi-tion of (sometimes poisonous) substances to food in the attempt to make it go further, look more attractive, to disguise spoilage or increase profits.[1] A chemist called Frederick Accum was one of the first to draw attention to this in his 1820 exposé *A Treatise on Adulteration of Food and Culinary Poisons*, in which he uncovered that toxic metals such as copper and lead were often used to change the colour of food. Green veg was made greener with copper, colourful sweets were made more vibrant with red lead, and fake tea was painted with oxidised copper to make it look more tea-like. These metals, being harmful at high doses, can cause stomach ache, nausea and organ damage. So it's thought this toxicity played a role in the high levels of industrial workers being off sick. Some decades later, other public health pioneers created extensive reports on what was going into food and the evidence that adulterated food was actually more commonplace than people believed led to the start of a long journey with many reforms to help protect us from these crooks.

If we dive into the food-labelling world today, we're presented with a lot of information. This is meant to be accurate, easy to understand and shouldn't be misleading. It also can't imply a food can prevent or treat a human disease. Let's unpick some of the terms, boxes and colour codes to make sense of what we see on our shop shelves.

Front of pack labelling

Front of pack labelling is also known as the traffic light labelling system, where calories, fat, sat fat, sugar and salt per portion or 100g are coded as green (low), amber (medium) and red (high). This method of food labelling is only voluntary, but many supermarkets and brands take part. The idea is that you can use it to quickly compare different food products, aiming to help you make an informed choice. This can also provide a percentage of the reference intake for that nutrient. The reference intake is not a target, but more of a guideline limit, based on an average-sized woman.

A word or warning from us: while food labels play a really important role from a safety point of view and are useful for those of us who need to eat more of or avoid certain nutrients for medical reasons, they shouldn't be seen as a sole marker of a food's healthfulness. They're more of a tool. Take cheese, for example. Looking at its traffic light label, we see red everywhere. Eek! It's being coded high for calories, saturated fat and salt, so it could be easy to get swept up by reductionist thinking and take this food to be unhealthy. But cheese is also high in protein, rich in calcium and a good source of dairy, making it incredibly healthy in many contexts. Front of pack labelling can help make comparisons but it has the risk of being over-simplistic and demonising.

Back of pack food labelling

Most food packets have to provide a nutrition label on the back. This must include:

	Typical value per 100g	Typical value per serving (g)
Energy kcal		
Fat		
Of which saturates		
Carbohydrates		
Of which sugars		
Protein		
Salt		

Calories

The calorie content in kcal or kJ can let you know what the energy content is of the food product.

Fat

The fat content of a food on the back of pack label contains both saturated and unsaturated fat.

- High fat = more than 17.5g of fat per 100g
- Low fat = 3g or less per 100g
- Fat free = 0.5g of fat or less per 100g or 100ml

Saturated fat

It's possible to work out how much of the product contains saturated fat (and from the remaining fat, unsaturated fat) by looking at the 'saturates' content.

- High = more than 5g of saturates per 100g
- Low = 1.5g of saturated or less per 100g

Sugar

- High = more than 22.5g of total sugars per 100g
- Low sugar = 5g of total sugars or less per 100g
- Medium would be somewhere in the middle of these two!

The ingredients list

Labels might also provide a list of ingredients. These would be listed in descending order of weight. This means the main ingredients in the food are at the start of the list.

Allergens

In the UK, we follow the European Union laws for labelling food allergens on food packaging. Packaged food sold in the UK therefore must clearly declare if foods contain one of the eight most common food allergens (which account for around 90 per cent of food allergies), as well as some of the less commonly encountered allergens, like sulphites. Labels must highlight allergens in **bold** in ingredients lists, and brands are encouraged to include an allergy advice statement which refers you to the allergens in the list. For non-packaged foods, like those in restaurants or cafes, foods should be identified as containing allergens in writing or by speaking to staff.

Allergens which must be identified in the EU are:

- Cereals containing gluten, namely: wheat (such as spelt and khorasan wheat), rye, barley, oats.
- Crustaceans, for example: prawns, crabs, lobster, crayfish.
- Eggs.
- Fish.
- Peanuts.
- Soya beans.
- Milk (including lactose).
- Nuts; namely almonds, hazelnuts, walnuts, cashews, pecan nuts, Brazil nuts, pistachio nuts, macadamia (or Queensland) nuts.
- Celery (including celeriac).
- Mustard.
- Sesame.
- Sulphur dioxide/sulphites, where added and at a level above 10mg/kg or 10mg/l in the finished product. This can be used as a preservative in dried fruit.
- Lupin, which includes lupin seeds and flour and can be found in types of bread, pastries and pasta.
- Molluscs, such as mussels, whelks, oysters, snails and squid.

Navigating free sugars from the nutrition label

You can find lots of useful information about the food you're eating by looking at the label. We often get asked about free sugars (the sugars added during processing) and if it's

▶

possible to figure out how much is in our food. Unfortunately this information is not on food labels as it's not possible for manufacturers to analyse if the sugar has been added, was occurring naturally or has combined with other ingredients in the cooking process.

Nutrition labels must provide information about total sugars (both the free sugars and naturally occurring sugars) listed per 100g of product. Some products will also have this listed per portion. As we are only given a total sugar value, working out how much free sugars are in foods like yoghurt (with naturally occurring lactose) or in cereals with dried fruit (with naturally occurring sugars) can be more difficult. However, the ingredients list is a good place to start as sugars added to a product must be included in the ingredients list.

Step 1) The ingredients list

The first place to see whether your food contains sugars is the ingredients list. Ingredients are listed in order of weight. This means that if you see sugar near the top of the list, the food is likely to be high in free sugars. Watch out for other words used to describe the sugars added to food and drinks, such as:

- Cane sugar.
- Honey.
- Brown sugar.
- High-fructose corn syrup.
- Fruit juice concentrate/purées.
- Corn syrup.
- Fructose.
- Sucrose.

▶

- Glucose.
- Crystalline sucrose.
- Nectars (such as blossom).
- Maple and agave syrups.
- Dextrose.
- Maltose.
- Molasses.
- Treacle.

Step 2) The back/side of pack information panel

Here is where you find a table with the main nutrients contained in your food per 100g/ml and portion. Sugar is listed as both carbohydrate (which includes starch as sugars) and 'of which sugars'. The 'of which sugars' label describes the total amount of sugars from all sources: free sugars, plus those from milk, and those present in fruit and vegetables. For example, plain yoghurt may contain as much as 8g per serving, but none of these are free sugars, as they all come from milk. The same applies to an individual portion of fruit; an apple might contain around 11g of total sugar, depending on its size, the variety and the stage of ripeness. However, sugar in fruit is not considered free sugar unless the fruit is juiced or puréed.

E numbers

These are additives that have been tested for their safety. They might be added to stop food going off, improve the flavour, texture or make it look more attractive.

Other information: nutrition and health claims

Any nutrition or health claims on a label should have first been authorised and listed on a special register which aims to make sure the claims are scientifically sound and not misleading.

A health claim is any statement on a label that suggests a food brings a health benefit, such as supporting the immune system or reducing fatigue. They also may need to have met certain conditions, for example, to make the claim that oat beta-glucans lower cholesterol, the food must contain 1g of beta-glucans per portion.

- 'Wheat bran fibre contributes to an increase in faecal bulk.'
- 'Calcium is needed for the maintenance of normal bones.'
- 'Potassium contributes to the maintenance of normal blood pressure.'
- 'Folate contributes to maternal tissue growth during pregnancy.'
- 'Vitamin C contributes to the reduction of tiredness and fatigue.'

A nutrition claim is any claims that suggests a food has beneficial nutritional properties due to its ingredients. Some examples are:

- 'Sugar free' (must contain less than 0.5g sugars per 100g).
- 'Low fat' (must contain less than 3g fat per 100g).
- 'High in fibre' (must contain at least 6g fibre per 100g).
- 'Source of vitamin D' (must contain at least 15 per cent of the RI for vitamin D per 100g).
- 'High protein' (must contain at least 20 per cent of its calories from protein).

Best-before and use-by dates

Use-by: This is to do with the food safety and is often labelled on things that can go off quickly, like meats and cheese. Something called the sell-by date is usually a few days before the use-by date, to give you enough time to eat the food after buying it. It's best to eat food before the use-by date to avoid food poisoning (thinking a food looks and smells ok is not a reliable method!).

Best-before: This is about the quality of the food. It's not necessarily dangerous to eat foods beyond this date (they're mostly canned or dry foods like biscuits) but the flavour, colour or texture might be a bit, meh.

Enrichment

Where nutrients which were lost during the processing of food have been added back.

Fortification

Where vitamins and minerals have been added into foods which didn't originally contain them. This is a useful way to improve the nutrition of a population. Some foods are fortified by law (like white bread with a range of vitamins) and others voluntarily (e.g. spreads and breakfast cereals).

Acknowledgements

A note from us

We wrote a book! However, we certainly didn't do it alone and there are lots of people we need to thank for their support and contributions.

First of all, an enormous thank you to our literary agent, Emma Finn, who took a risk on us and made this book happen. We are so grateful for you. The guidance and support you offered us throughout this process was invaluable, we literally couldn't have done it without you. Thank you so much.

Special thanks to our fantastic editor, Jillian Young, for your patience, expertise and belief that people might buy a nutrition book based on balance and reason (in a time when quick fixes and fads still seem to rule). Also to Anna Steadman, for stepping in and taking such great care of us during Jillian's maternity leave, you helped us shape this book and make it so much better than we could have imagined – huge thanks to you, and everyone else at Piatkus who worked to bring this book to life.

A big thank you to John Ratford, our talented illustrator. We knew the moment we met that we wanted to work with you. You've always been so professional, getting images back to us in a flash and helping us convey some tricky nutrition concepts creatively.

A massive thank you to Captain Science for fact checking our work. We are so lucky to have had access to such a brilliant mind. Thanks for holding us to account and challenging us during the editing process. Your attention to detail made this book the best it could be.

As you may have realised, nutrition is complex! So we also need to say a big thank you to all the people who took the time to speak with us during the research process and who helped us to refine our understanding of the more tricky areas of the science, some of whom also contributed to this book; Alan Flanagan, Tom Butler, Duane Mellor, Sarah Dempster, Catherine Collins, Maeve Hanan, Andrea Davis, Helen MacLaughlin, James Wong, James Stewart, Ruairi Robertson, Alex Garzolla and Anthony Warner – thank you!

To the awesome, talented group of peers who have supported us professionally and personally since we set up at The Rooted Project; Laura Thomas, Megan Rossi, Nichola Whitehead, you rock! Thanks for being there for us, for your contributions to this book, but most of all for the tireless work you do in promoting evidence and reason in a field fraught with fads and nonsense.

A note from Rosie

At the end of writing this book, my baby Enzo was diagnosed with a rare, aggressive form of infant leukaemia at the age of one. It was a big shock to us all and has quite literally turned our lives upside down. Helen, being an amazing friend and colleague, was beyond supportive – taking the reins without question and quietly battling in the background to meet final deadlines. Alongside managing to do some late-night tinkering beside the hospital bed, Helen has never put an ounce of pressure on me to do more than I can, despite being under immense stress herself. Life affirming experiences often confirm what's important. For me it's family, friends and doing what I love. Thank you, Helen, for playing a big part in this.

I also want to thank my husband Ant. Part of the reason why I love food as much as I do is down to you. You were cheering me on from the sidelines when I decided to re-train in dietetics (I promise I won't become a student again for a while) and the past decade together has been filled with such memorable mealtime moments. You've also been the most solid of rocks throughout this book writing process. Getting pen to paper with a newborn who doesn't sleep is hard, but you made it manageable. When Enzo was six months old, you had a month off between jobs and made it your mission to give me as much writing time as possible. While you boys threw yourselves into soft play, scenic walks and other sensory experiences, I could capture generous windows of time to write. This was gold dust. I'm so lucky to have you in my life and love you more every day.

Thank you to all my amazing wider family – Mum, Dad, Max, Kitty, Alice and my mother-in-law Maria – and friends for supporting me and acting as critical sounding boards over and over again. You came up with some more than imaginative book name options over wine and cheese (*The Food, The Fads and The Fugly* sadly didn't make the cut) and I'm so lucky to have such a generous, thoughtful, fun group of people in my life. Thank you for always being there for me.

And finally Enzo. Thank you for making me laugh until my sides hurt over this past year. Your sense of humour is contagious and your love has kept me going. You're really quite amazing.

A note from Helen

Writing a book is hard (who knew?!) and so I need to start by saying a huge thank you to Rosie. Working with you is always a total dream and I couldn't have hoped for a better partner in crime for this book, or The Rooted Project. I'm not sure I would have been as awesome as you, during this writing process, were it me juggling writing with a newborn baby as a sleep deprived first-time mum. You have handled everything, even the awful challenges of the last few months, with strength and grace. Thank you for all your hard work. You really are the best.

I also want to say a huge thank you to my husband Jim. Juggling military and family life can be hard, but you take everything in your stride. Thank you for giving me the space and time to write, even when it meant sacrificing precious time with you and our boy while you were at home. Thank you for everything you do, but most of all for being the best dad and husband I could wish for. Austin and I are so lucky to have you and we both love you loads.

To my amazing wider family (Peter, Dan, Laura, Ian, Amy and the minis, Oliver and Anabelle); thank you for putting up with me, I love you all lots and am so lucky to have you in my corner cheering me on. Special thanks to my mum and dad, Maureen and Nigel, and my mother and father-in-law, Helen and Steve, for all the babysitting and support while Jim was away overseas.

An extra thank you to Laura Thomas from me (you got two!) for all the pep talks and support you gave while I was writing this book. You had all kinds of other stuff going on, but always made time to provide words of encouragement and wisdom. I'm so lucky that I can call you my friend.

And finally, a huge thank you to the tiny jam monster in my life, Austin. Your smile, laugh and sense of humour light up my world. I love you the most. Don't tell Dad.

References

Chapter 1 What's the Harm?

1 Liese, A. D., Krebs-Smith, S. M., Subar, A. F., George, S. M., Harmon, B. E., Neuhouser, M. L., Boushey, C. J., Schap, T. E. and Reedy, J. (2015) 'The Dietary Patterns Methods Project: Synthesis of Findings across Cohorts and Relevance to Dietary Guidance', The Journal of Nutrition, 145(3), pp. 393–402. doi: 10.3945/jn.114.205336.

2 Onvani, S., Haghighatdoost, F., Surkan, P. J., Larijani, B. and Azadbakht, L. (2017) 'Adherence to the Healthy Eating Index and Alternative Healthy Eating Index dietary patterns and mortality from all causes, cardiovascular disease and cancer: a meta-analysis of observational studies', Journal of Human Nutrition and Dietetics, 30(2), pp. 216–226. doi: 10.1111/jhn.12415.

3 www.mintel.com/press-centre/social-and-lifestyle/ vitamin-and-supplements-market-in-good-health-46-of-all-brits-are-daily-users – Google Search (no date). Available at: https://www.google. com/search?client=safari&rls=en&q=www.mintel.com/press-centre/ social-and-lifestyle/vitamin-and-supplements-market-in-good-health-46-of-all-brits-are-daily-users&ie=UTF-8&oe=UTF-8 (Accessed: 8 March 2019).

4 Alexander, D. D., Weed, D. L., Chang, E. T., Miller, P. E., Mohamed, M. A. and Elkayam, L. (2013) 'A Systematic Review of Multivitamin– Multimineral Use and Cardiovascular Disease and Cancer Incidence and Total Mortality', Journal of the American College of Nutrition, 32(5), pp. 339–354. doi: 10.1080/07315724.2013.839909.

5 Vici, G., Belli, L., Biondi, M. and Polzonetti, V. (2016) 'Gluten free

diet and nutrient deficiencies: A review', Clinical Nutrition, 35(6), pp. 1236–1241. doi:10.1016/j.clnu.2016.05.002.

6 Staudacher, H. M. (2017) 'Nutritional, microbiological and psychosocial implications of the low FODMAP diet', Journal of Gastroenterology and Hepatology. John Wiley & Sons, Ltd (10.1111), 32, pp. 16–19. doi: 10.1111/jgh.13688.

7 Koven, N. S. and Abry, A. W. (2015) 'The clinical basis of orthorexia nervosa: emerging perspectives.', Neuropsychiatric disease and treatment. Dove Press, 11, pp. 385–94. doi: 10.2147/NDT.S61665.

8 https://academic.oup.com/jnci/article-abstract/110/1/ djx145/4064136/Use-of-Alternative-Medicine-for-Cancer-and-Its?redirectedFrom=fulltext

9 Tartaglia, S. and Rollero, C. (2015) 'The Effects of Attractiveness and Status on Personality Evaluation.', Europe's journal of psychology. PsychOpen, 11(4), pp. 677–90. doi: 10.5964/ejop.v11i4.896.

Chapter 2 Calories

1 Raichle, M. E. and Gusnard, D. A. (2002) 'Appraising the brain's energy budget.', Proceedings of the National Academy of Sciences of the United States of America. National Academy of Sciences, 99(16), pp. 10237–9. doi: 10.1073/pnas.172399499.

2 Mergenthaler, P., Lindauer, U., Dienel, G. A. and Meisel, A. (2013) 'Sugar for the brain: the role of glucose in physiological and pathological brain function.', Trends in neurosciences. NIH Public Access, 36(10), pp. 587–97. doi: 10.1016/j.tins.2013.07.001.

3 Hall, K. D., Heymsfield, S. B., Kemnitz, J. W., Klein, S., Schoeller, D. A. and Speakman, J. R. (2012) 'Energy balance and its components: implications for body weight regulation.', The American journal of clinical nutrition. American Society for Nutrition, 95(4), pp. 989–94. doi: 10.3945/ajcn.112.036350.

4 Dulloo, A. G., Geissler, C. A., Horton, T., Collins, A. and Miller, D. S. (1989) 'Normal caffeine consumption: influence on thermogenesis and daily energy expenditure in lean and postobese human volunteers', The American Journal of Clinical Nutrition, 49(1), pp. 44–50. doi: 10.1093/ajcn/49.1.44.

5 Thielecke, F., Rahn, G., Böhnke, J., Adams, F., Birkenfeld, A. L., Jordan, J. and Boschmann, M. (2010) 'Epigallocatechin-3-gallate and postprandial fat oxidation in overweight/obese male volunteers: a pilot study', European Journal of Clinical Nutrition, 64(7), pp. 704–713. doi: 10.1038/ejcn.2010.47.

6 Lonac, M. C., Richards, J. C., Schweder, M. M., Johnson, T. K. and

Bell, C. (2011) 'Influence of Short-Term Consumption of the Caffeine-Free, Epigallocatechin-3-Gallate Supplement, Teavigo, on Resting Metabolism and the Thermic Effect of Feeding', Obesity, 19(2), pp. 298–304. doi: 10.1038/oby.2010.181.

7   First manslaughter conviction for DNP diet pill dealer after toxic pills killed student (no date). Available at: https://www.telegraph.co.uk/news/2018/06/27/first-manslaughter-conviction-dnp-diet-pilldealer-toxic-pills/ (Accessed: 8 March 2019).

8   Hall, K. D., Heymsfield, S. B., Kemnitz, J. W., Klein, S., Schoeller, D. A. and Speakman, J. R. (2012) 'Energy balance and its components: implications for body weight regulation.', The American journal of clinical nutrition. American Society for Nutrition, 95(4), pp. 989–94. doi: 10.3945/ajcn.112.036350.

9   Childs, E. and de Wit, H. (2006) 'Subjective, behavioral, and physiological effects of acute caffeine in light, nondependent caffeine users', Psychopharmacology, 185(4), pp. 514–523. doi: 10.1007/s00213-006-0341-3.

10 Howell, L. L. and Byrd, L. D. (1993) 'Effects of CGS 15943, a nonxanthine adenosine antagonist, on behavior in the squirrel monkey.', The Journal of pharmacology and experimental therapeutics, 267(1), pp. 432–9. Available at: http://www.ncbi.nlm.nih.gov/pubmed/8229772 (Accessed: 8 March 2019).

11 Haskell, C. F., Kennedy, D. O., Wesnes, K. A. and Scholey, A. B. (2005) 'Cognitive and mood improvements of caffeine in habitual consumers and habitual non-consumers of caffeine', Psychopharmacology, 179(4), pp. 813–825. doi: 10.1007/s00213-004-2104-3.

12 Müller, M. J. and Bosy-Westphal, A. (2013) 'Adaptive thermogenesis with weight loss in humans', Obesity. John Wiley & Sons, Ltd, 21(2), pp. 218–228. doi: 10.1002/oby.20027.

13 Polidori, D., Sanghvi, A., Seeley, R. J. and Hall, K. D. (2016) 'How Strongly Does Appetite Counter Weight Loss? Quantification of the Feedback Control of Human Energy Intake', Obesity, 24(11), pp. 2289–2295. doi: 10.1002/oby.21653.

14 Anderson, J. W., Konz, E. C., Frederich, R. C. and Wood, C. L. (2001) 'Long-term weight-loss maintenance: a meta-analysis of US studies', The American Journal of Clinical Nutrition, 74(5), pp. 579–584. doi: 10.1093/ajcn/74.5.579.

15 Oike, H., Oishi, K. and Kobori, M. (2014) 'Nutrients, Clock Genes, and Chrononutrition.', Current nutrition reports. Springer, 3(3), pp. 204–212. doi: 10.1007/s13668-014-0082-6.

16 Froy, O. (2010) 'Metabolism and Circadian Rhythms—Implications for Obesity', Endocrine Reviews, 31(1), pp. 1–24. doi: 10.1210/er.2009-0014.

17 Marcheva, B., Ramsey, K. M., Peek, C. B., Affinati, A., Maury, E. and Bass, J. (2013) 'Circadian clocks and metabolism.', Handbook of experimental pharmacology. NIH Public Access, (217), pp. 127–55. doi: 10.1007/978-3-642-25950-0_6.

18 James, S. M., Honn, K. A., Gaddameedhi, S. and Van Dongen, H. P. A. (2017) 'Shift Work: Disrupted Circadian Rhythms and Sleep-Implications for Health and Well-Being.', Current sleep medicine reports. NIH Public Access, 3(2), pp. 104–112. doi:10.1007/s40675-017-0071-6.

19 Solbrig, L., Jones, R., Kavanagh, D., May, J., Parkin, T. and Andrade, J. (2017) 'People trying to lose weight dislike calorie counting apps and want motivational support to help them achieve their goals.', Internet interventions. Elsevier, 7, pp. 23–31. doi:10.1016/j.invent.2016.12.003.

20 Use, Evidence and Remaining Barriers to Mainstream Acceptance Patient Adoption of mHealth (2015). Available at: www.theimsinstitute.org (Accessed: 8 March 2019).

21 Zhao, J., Freeman, B. and Li, M. (2016) 'Can Mobile Phone Apps Influence People's Health Behavior Change? An Evidence Review.', Journal of medical Internet research. Journal of Medical Internet Research, 18(11), p. e287. doi: 10.2196/jmir.5692.

22 McKay, F. H., Cheng, C., Wright, A., Shill, J., Stephens, H. and Uccellini, M. (2018) 'Evaluating mobile phone applications for health behaviour change: A systematic review', Journal of Telemedicine and Telecare, 24(1), pp. 22–30. doi:10.1177/1357633X16673538.

23 Davis, S. F., Ellsworth, M. A., Payne, H. E., Hall, S. M., West, J. H. and Nordhagen, A. L. (2016) 'Health Behavior Theory in Popular Calorie Counting Apps: A Content Analysis.', JMIR mHealth and uHealth. JMIR Publications Inc., 4(1), p. e19. doi:10.2196/mhealth.4177.

24 Bardus, M., van Beurden, S. B., Smith, J. R. and Abraham, C. (2016) 'A review and content analysis of engagement, functionality, aesthetics, information quality, and change techniques in the most popular commercial apps for weight management', International Journal of Behavioral Nutrition and Physical Activity, 13(1), p. 35. doi:10.1186/s12966-016-0359-9.

25 Rivera, J., McPherson, A., Hamilton, J., Birken, C., Coons, M., Iyer, S., Agarwal, A., Lalloo, C. and Stinson, J. (2016) 'Mobile Apps for Weight Management: A Scoping Review.', JMIR mHealth and uHealth. JMIR Publications Inc., 4(3), p. e87. doi:10.2196/mhealth.5115.

26 Simpson, C. C. and Mazzeo, S. E. (2017) 'Calorie counting and fitness tracking technology: Associations with eating disorder symptomatology', Eating Behaviors, 26, pp. 89–92. doi: 10.1016/j. eatbeh.2017.02.002.

27 Levinson, C. A., Fewell, L. and Brosof, L. C. (2017) 'My Fitness Pal calorie tracker usage in the eating disorders', Eating Behaviors, 27, pp. 14–16. doi:10.1016/j.eatbeh.2017.08.003.

28 Simpson, C. C. and Mazzeo, S. E. (2017) 'Calorie counting and fitness tracking technology: Associations with eating disorder symptomatology', Eating Behaviors. Pergamon, 26, pp. 89–92. doi: 10.1016/J.EATBEH.2017.02.002.

29 Hilbert, A., Pike, K. M., Goldschmidt, A. B., Wilfley, D. E., Fairburn, C. G., Dohm, F.-A., Walsh, B. T. and Striegel Weissman, R. (2014) 'Risk factors across the eating disorders.', Psychiatry research. NIH Public Access, 220(1–2), pp. 500–6. doi:10.1016/j.psychres.2014.05.054.

30 Eikey, E. V., Reddy, M. C., Booth, K. M., Kvasny, L., Blair, J. L., Li, V. and Poole, E. S. (2017) 'Desire to Be Underweight: Exploratory Study on a Weight Loss App Community and User Perceptions of the Impact on Disordered Eating Behaviors.', JMIR mHealth and uHealth. JMIR Publications Inc., 5(10), p. e150. doi: 10.2196/mhealth.6683.

31 Simpson, C. C. and Mazzeo, S. E. (2017) 'Calorie counting and fitness tracking technology: Associations with eating disorder symptomatology', Eating Behaviors, 26, pp. 89–92. doi: 10.1016/j. eatbeh.2017.02.002

32 Davidsen, L., Vistisen, B. and Astrup, A. (2007) 'Impact of the menstrual cycle on determinants of energy balance: a putative role in weight loss attempts', International Journal of Obesity, 31(12), pp. 1777–1785. doi: 10.1038/sj.ijo.0803699.

Chapter 3 Fats

1 Saturated fats and heart disease link 'unproven' - NHS (no date). Available at: https://www.nhs.uk/news/heart-and-lungs/saturated-fats-and-heart-disease-link-unproven/ (Accessed: 8 March 2019).

2 (no date). Available at: http://www.truehealthinitiative.org/wordpress/wp-content/uploads/2017/07/ (Accessed: 8 March 2019).

3 Fan, J., Kitajima, S., Watanabe, T., Xu, J., Zhang, J., Liu, E. and Chen, Y. E. (2015) 'Rabbit models for the study of human atherosclerosis: from pathophysiological mechanisms to translational medicine.', Pharmacology & therapeutics. NIH Public Access, 146, pp. 104–19. doi: 10.1016/j.pharmthera.2014.09.009.

4 Wong, B., Kruse, G., Kutikova, L., Ray, K. K., Mata, P. and Bruckert, E. (2016) 'Cardiovascular Disease Risk Associated With Familial Hypercholesterolemia: A Systematic Review of the Literature', Clinical Therapeutics, 38(7), pp. 1696–1709. doi:10.1016/j.clinthera.2016.05.006.

5 Biggerstaff, K. D. and Wooten, J. S. (2004) 'Understanding lipoproteins as transporters of cholesterol and other lipids', Advances in Physiology Education, 28(3), pp. 105–106. doi: 10.1152/advan.00048.2003.

6 Zewinger, S., Drechsler, C., Kleber, M. E., Dressel, A., Riffel, J., Triem, S., Lehmann, M., Kopecky, C., Säemann, M. D., Lepper, P. M., Silbernagel, G., Scharnagl, H., Ritsch, A., Thorand, B., de las Heras Gala, T., Wagenpfeil, S., Koenig, W., Peters, A., Laufs, U., Wanner, C., Fliser, D., Speer, T. and März, W. (2015) 'Serum amyloid A: high-density lipoproteins interaction and cardiovascular risk', European Heart Journal, 36(43), p. ehv352. doi: 10.1093/eurheartj/ehv352.

7 Moriyama, K. and Takahashi, E. (2016) 'Non-HDL Cholesterol is a More Superior Predictor of Small-Dense LDL Cholesterol than LDL Cholesterol in Japanese Subjects with TG Levels <400 mg/dL', Journal of Atherosclerosis and Thrombosis, 23(9), pp. 1126–1137. doi: 10.5551/jat.33985.

8 Wang, T. D., Chen, W. J., Chien, K. L., Seh-Yi Su, S. S., Hsu, H. C., Chen, M. F., Liau, C. S. and Lee, Y. T. (2001) 'Efficacy of cholesterol levels and ratios in predicting future coronary heart disease in a Chinese population.', The American journal of cardiology, 88(7), pp. 737–43. Available at: http://www.ncbi.nlm.nih.gov/pubmed/11589839 (Accessed: 8 March 2019).

9 Gaziano, J. M., Hennekens, C. H., O'Donnell, C. J., Breslow, J. L. and Buring, J. E. (1997) 'Fasting triglycerides, high-density lipoprotein, and risk of myocardial infarction.', Circulation, 96(8), pp. 2520–5. Available at: http://www.ncbi.nlm.nih.gov/pubmed/9355888 (Accessed: 8 March 2019).

10 Shortreed, S. M., Peeters, A. and Forbes, A. B. (2013) 'Estimating the effect of long-term physical activity on cardiovascular disease and mortality: evidence from the Framingham Heart Study', Heart, 99(9), pp. 649–654. doi: 10.1136/heartjnl-2012-303461.

11 1980s fat guidelines 'lacked evidence,' study argues – NHS (no date). Available at: https://www.nhs.uk/news/food-and-diet/1980s-fat-guidelines-lacked-evidence-study-argues/ (Accessed: 8 March 2019).

12 Mozaffarian, D., Rosenberg, I. and Uauy, R. (2018) 'History of modern nutrition science-implications for current research, dietary guidelines, and food policy.', BMJ (Clinical research ed.). British Medical Journal Publishing Group, 361, p. k2392. doi:10.1136/bmj.k2392.

13 Facts and figures - Information for journalists - BHF (no date).
    Available at: https://www.bhf.org.uk/for-professionals/press-centre/
    facts-and-figures (Accessed: 8 March 2019).

14 Number of people living with diabetes doubles in twenty years |
    Diabetes UK (no date). Available at: https://www.diabetes.org.uk/About_
    us/News/diabetes-prevalence-statistics (Accessed: 8 March 2019).

15 Hu, F. B. (2010) 'Are refined carbohydrates worse than saturated fat?',
    The American Journal of Clinical Nutrition, 91(6), pp. 1541–1542. doi:
    10.3945/ajcn.2010.29622.

16 Siri-Tarino, P. W., Sun, Q., Hu, F. B. and Krauss, R. M. (2010) 'Meta-
    analysis of prospective cohort studies evaluating the association of
    saturated fat with cardiovascular disease', The American Journal of
    Clinical Nutrition, 91(3), pp. 535–546. doi:10.3945/ajcn.2009.27725.

17 Jakobsen, M. U., O'Reilly, E. J., Heitmann, B. L., Pereira, M. A.,
    Bälter, K., Fraser, G. E., Goldbourt, U., Hallmans, G., Knekt, P., Liu,
    S., Pietinen, P., Spiegelman, D., Stevens, J., Virtamo, J., Willett, W. C.
    and Ascherio, A. (2009) 'Major types of dietary fat and risk of coronary
    heart disease: a pooled analysis of 11 cohort studies', The American
    Journal of Clinical Nutrition, 89(5), pp. 1425–1432. doi: 10.3945/
    ajcn.2008.27124.

18 Jakobsen, M. U., Dethlefsen, C., Joensen, A. M., Stegger, J.,
    Tjønneland, A., Schmidt, E. B. and Overvad, K. (2010) 'Intake of
    carbohydrates compared with intake of saturated fatty acids and
    risk of myocardial infarction: importance of the glycemic index',
    The American Journal of Clinical Nutrition, 91(6), pp. 1764–1768.
    doi:10.3945/ajcn.2009.29099.

19 Drouin-Chartier, J.-P., Brassard, D., Tessier-Grenier, M., Côté, J.
    A., Labonté, M.-È., Desroches, S., Couture, P. and Lamarche, B.
    (2016) 'Systematic Review of the Association between Dairy Product
    Consumption and Risk of Cardiovascular-Related Clinical Outcomes.',
    Advances in nutrition (Bethesda, Md.). American Society for Nutrition,
    7(6), pp. 1026–1040. doi: 10.3945/an.115.011403.

20 Smoczyn'ski, M., Staniewski, B. and Kiełczewska, K. (2012)
    'Composition and Structure of the Bovine Milk Fat Globule
    Membrane—Some Nutritional and Technological Implications', Food
    Reviews International. Taylor & Francis Group , 28(2), pp. 188–202.
    doi: 10.1080/87559129.2011.595024.

21 Rosqvist, F., Smedman, A., Lindmark-Månsson, H., Paulsson, M.,
    Petrus, P., Straniero, S., Rudling, M., Dahlman, I. and Risérus, U.
    (2015) 'Potential role of milk fat globule membrane in modulating

plasma lipoproteins, gene expression, and cholesterol metabolism in humans: a randomized study', The American Journal of Clinical Nutrition, 102(1), pp. 20–30. doi: 10.3945/ajcn.115.107045.

22 Thorning, T. K., Bertram, H. C., Bonjour, J.-P., de Groot, L., Dupont, D., Feeney, E., Ipsen, R., Lecerf, J. M., Mackie, A., McKinley, M. C., Michalski, M.-C., Rémond, D., Risérus, U., Soedamah-Muthu, S. S., Tholstrup, T., Weaver, C., Astrup, A. and Givens, I. (2017) 'Whole dairy matrix or single nutrients in assessment of health effects: current evidence and knowledge gaps', The American Journal of Clinical Nutrition, 105(5), pp. 1033–1045. doi: 10.3945/ajcn.116.151548.

23 Mozaffarian, D. (2011) 'The Great Fat Debate: Taking the Focus Off of Saturated Fat', Journal of the American Dietetic Association, 111(5), pp. 665–666. doi:10.1016/j.jada.2011.03.030.

24 Sacks, F. M., Lichtenstein, A. H., Wu, J. H. Y., Appel, L. J., Creager, M. A., Kris-Etherton, P. M., Miller, M., Rimm, E. B., Rudel, L. L., Robinson, J. G., Stone, N. J. and Van Horn, L. V. (2017) 'Dietary Fats and Cardiovascular Disease: A Presidential Advisory From the American Heart Association', Circulation, 136(3). doi:10.1161/CIR.0000000000000510.

25 R. A McCance, AFRC Institute of Food Research, Public Health England, R. S. of C. (Great B. (issuing body) (2014) McCance and Widdowson's the Composition of Foods. 7th edn. RSC.

26 Mozaffarian, D., Aro, A. and Willett, W. C. (2009) 'Health effects of trans-fatty acids: experimental and observational evidence', European Journal of Clinical Nutrition, 63(S2), pp. S5–S21. doi: 10.1038/sj.ejcn.1602973.

27 NDNS: results from years 7 and 8 (combined) - GOV.UK (no date). Available at: https://www.gov.uk/government/statistics/ndns-results-from-years-7-and-8-combined (Accessed: 8 March 2019).

28 Lockyer, S. and Stanner, S. (2016) 'Coconut oil - a nutty idea?', Nutrition Bulletin, 41(1), pp. 42–54. doi: 10.1111/nbu.12188.

29 Clegg, M. E. (2017) 'They say coconut oil can aid weight loss, but can it really?', European Journal of Clinical Nutrition, 71(10), pp. 1139–1143. doi:10.1038/ejcn.2017.86.

30 Clegg, M. E. (2017) 'They say coconut oil can aid weight loss, but can it really?', European Journal of Clinical Nutrition, 71(10), pp. 1139–1143. doi:10.1038/ejcn.2017.86.

31 Sacks, F. M., Lichtenstein, A. H., Wu, J. H. Y., Appel, L. J., Creager, M. A., Kris-Etherton, P. M., Miller, M., Rimm, E. B., Rudel, L. L., Robinson, J. G., Stone, N. J., Van Horn, L. V. and American

Heart Association (2017) 'Dietary Fats and Cardiovascular Disease: A Presidential Advisory From the American Heart Association', Circulation, 136(3), pp. e1–e23. doi: 10.1161/CIR.0000000000000510.

32 Sacks, F. M., Lichtenstein, A. H., Wu, J. H. Y., Appel, L. J., Creager, M. A., Kris-Etherton, P. M., Miller, M., Rimm, E. B., Rudel, L. L., Robinson, J. G., Stone, N. J., Van Horn, L. V. and American Heart Association (2017) 'Dietary Fats and Cardiovascular Disease: A Presidential Advisory From the American Heart Association', Circulation, 136(3), pp. e1–e23. doi: 10.1161/CIR.0000000000000510.

Chapter 4 Carbohydrates

1 Heart Disease and Diabetes Risks Tied to Carbs, Not Fat, Study Finds (no date). Available at: https://www.livescience.com/48969-heart-disease-diabetes-risks-carbohydrate-saturated-fat.html (Accessed: 8 March 2019).

2 'Carbs linked to lung cancer,' study finds - NHS (no date). Available at: https://www.nhs.uk/news/cancer/carbs-linked-to-lung-cancer-study-finds/ (Accessed: 8 March 2019).

3 Hall, K. D. and Guo, J. (2017) 'Obesity Energetics: Body Weight Regulation and the Effects of Diet Composition.', Gastroenterology. NIH Public Access, 152(7), p.1718–1727.e3. doi: 10.1053/j.gastro.2017.01.052.Leaf, A. and Antonio, J. (2017) 'The Effects of Overfeeding on Body Composition: The Role of Macronutrient Composition – A Narrative Review.', International journal of exercise science. Western Kentucky University, 10(8), pp. 1275–1296. Available at: http://www.ncbi.nlm.nih.gov/pubmed/29399253 (Accessed: 8 March 2019).

4 Leaf, A. and Antonio, J. (2017) 'The Effects of Overfeeding on Body Composition: The Role of Macronutrient Composition - A Narrative Review.', International journal of exercise science. Western Kentucky University, 10(8), pp. 1275–1296. Available at: http://www.ncbi.nlm.nih.gov/pubmed/29399253 (Accessed: 8 March 2019).

5 Obesity System Influence Diagram (no date). Available at: http://www.shiftn.com/obesity/Full-Map.html (Accessed: 8 March 2019).

6 Drummen, M., Tischmann, L., Gatta-Cherifi, B., Adam, T. and Westerterp-Plantenga, M. (2018) 'Dietary Protein and Energy Balance in Relation to Obesity and Co-morbidities.', Frontiers in endocrinology. Frontiers Media SA, 9, p. 443. doi:10.3389/fendo.2018.00443.

7 Kreitzman, S. N., Coxon, A. Y. and Szaz, K. F. (1992) 'Glycogen storage: illusions of easy weight loss, excessive weight regain, and

distortions in estimates of body composition', The American Journal of Clinical Nutrition, 56(1), p. 292S–293S. doi:10.1093/ajcn/56.1.292S.

8　Kreitzman, S. N., Coxon, A. Y. and Szaz, K. F. (1992) 'Glycogen storage: illusions of easy weight loss, excessive weight regain, and distortions in estimates of body composition', The American Journal of Clinical Nutrition, 56(1), p. 292S–293S. doi:10.1093/ajcn/56.1.292S.

9　Gardner, C. D., Trepanowski, J. F., Del Gobbo, L. C., Hauser, M. E., Rigdon, J., Ioannidis, J. P. A., Desai, M. and King, A. C. (2018) 'Effect of Low-Fat vs Low-Carbohydrate Diet on 12-Month Weight Loss in Overweight Adults and the Association With Genotype Pattern or Insulin Secretion', JAMA, 319(7), p. 667. doi:10.1001/jama.2018.0245.

10　Hall, K. D. and Kahan, S. (2018) 'Maintenance of Lost Weight and Long-Term Management of Obesity', Medical Clinics of North America, 102(1), pp. 183–197. doi:10.1016/j.mcna.2017.08.012.

11　Gardner, C. D., Trepanowski, J. F., Del Gobbo, L. C., Hauser, M. E., Rigdon, J., Ioannidis, J. P. A., Desai, M. and King, A. C. (2018) 'Effect of Low-Fat vs Low-Carbohydrate Diet on 12-Month Weight Loss in Overweight Adults and the Association With Genotype Pattern or Insulin Secretion', JAMA, 319(7), p. 667. doi:10.1001/jama.2018.0245.

12　Schwartz, M. W., Seeley, R. J., Zeltser, L. M., Drewnowski, A., Ravussin, E., Redman, L. M. and Leibel, R. L. (2017) 'Obesity Pathogenesis: An Endocrine Society Scientific Statement', Endocrine Reviews. Oxford University Press, 38(4), pp. 267–296. doi:10.1210/er.2017-00111.

13　Hardy, K., Brand-Miller, J., Brown, K. D., Thomas, M. G. and Copeland, L. (2015) 'THE IMPORTANCE OF DIETARY CARBOHYDRATE IN HUMAN EVOLUTION.', The Quarterly review of biology, 90(3), pp. 251–68. Available at: http://www.ncbi.nlm.nih.gov/pubmed/26591850 (Accessed: 8 March 2019).

14　Teo, K., Chow, C. K., Vaz, M., Rangarajan, S., Yusuf, S. and PURE Investigators-Writing Group (2009) 'The Prospective Urban Rural Epidemiology (PURE) study: Examining the impact of societal influences on chronic noncommunicable diseases in low-, middle-, and high-income countries', American Heart Journal, 158(1), p. 1–7.e1. doi:10.1016/j.ahj.2009.04.019.

15　Low-carb diets could shorten life, study suggests - BBC News (no date). Available at: https://www.bbc.co.uk/news/health-45195474 (Accessed: 8 March 2019).

16　Low-fat diets could kill you, shows major study | The Independent (no date). Available at: https://www.independent.co.uk/life-style/

health-and-families/low-fat-diets-kill-you-study-food-drink-eat-health-barcelona-cardiology-canada-a7918666.html (Accessed: 8 March 2019).

17 Great Britain. Scientific Advisory Committee on Nutrition. and Stationery Office (Great Britain) (no date) Carbohydrates and health. Available at: https://www.gov.uk/government/publications/sacn-carbohydrates-and-health-report (Accessed: 8 March 2019).

18 NDNS: results from years 7 and 8 (combined) – GOV.UK (no date). Available at: https://www.gov.uk/government/statistics/ndns-results-from-years-7-and-8-combined (Accessed: 8 March 2019).

19 van der Kamp, J. W., Poutanen, K., Seal, C. J. and Richardson, D. P. (2014) 'The HEALTHGRAIN definition of "whole grain"', Food & Nutrition Research, 58(1), p. 22100. doi: 10.3402/fnr.v58.22100.

20 Mozaffarian, R. S., Lee, R. M., Kennedy, M. A., Ludwig, D. S., Mozaffarian, D. and Gortmaker, S. L. (2013) 'Identifying whole grain foods: a comparison of different approaches for selecting more healthful whole grain products', Public Health Nutrition, 16(12), pp. 2255–2264. doi: 10.1017/S1368980012005447.

21 Zong, G., Gao, A., Hu, F. B. and Sun, Q. (2016) 'Whole Grain Intake and Mortality From All Causes, Cardiovascular Disease, and Cancer', Circulation. Lippincott Williams & Wilkins Hagerstown, MD , 133(24), pp. 2370–2380. doi:10.1161/CIRCULATIONAHA.115.021101.

22 Lang, R. and Jebb, S. A. (2019) 'Who consumes whole grains, and how much?', Proceedings of the Nutrition Society, 62, pp. 123–127. doi: 10.1079/PNS2002219.

23 Mozaffarian, R. S., Lee, R. M., Kennedy, M. A., Ludwig, D. S., Mozaffarian, D. and Gortmaker, S. L. (2013) 'Identifying whole grain foods: a comparison of different approaches for selecting more healthful whole grain products', Public Health Nutrition, 16(12), pp. 2255–2264. doi: 10.1017/S1368980012005447.

Chapter 5 Sugar

1 Children in England consuming 'twice as much sugar as recommended' – BBC News (no date). Available at: https://www.bbc.co.uk/news/health-44483081 (Accessed: 8 March 2019).

2 Action on Sugar – Action on Sugar (no date). Available at: http://www.actiononsugar.org/ (Accessed: 8 March 2019).

3 Reducing Sugar | Cutting Out Sugar | Change4Life (no date). Available at: https://www.nhs.uk/change4life/food-facts/sugar (Accessed: 8 March 2019).

4 Mozaffarian, D., Rosenberg, I. and Uauy, R. (2018) 'History of modern nutrition science-implications for current research, dietary guidelines, and food policy.', BMJ (Clinical research ed.). British Medical Journal Publishing Group, 361, p. k2392. doi:10.1136/bmj.k2392.

5 The sugar conspiracy – The Telegraph (no date). Available at: https://www.theguardian.com/society/2016/apr/07/the-sugar-conspiracy-robert-lustig-john-yudkin

6 Oldways Common Ground Consensus | Oldways (no date). Available at: https://oldwayspt.org/programs/oldways-common-ground/oldways-common-ground-consensus (Accessed: 8 March 2019).

7 Wang, X., Ouyang, Y., Liu, J., Zhu, M., Zhao, G., Bao, W. and Hu, F. B. (2014) 'Fruit and vegetable consumption and mortality from all causes, cardiovascular disease, and cancer: systematic review and dose-response meta-analysis of prospective cohort studies', BMJ, 349(jul29 3), pp. g4490–g4490. doi: 10.1136/bmj.g4490.

8 Christensen, A. S., Viggers, L., Hasselström, K. and Gregersen, S. (2013) 'Effect of fruit restriction on glycemic control in patients with type 2 diabetes--a randomized trial.', Nutrition journal. BioMed Central, 12, p. 29. doi: 10.1186/1475-2891-12-29.

9 NDNS: results from years 7 and 8 (combined) – GOV.UK (no date). Available at: https://www.gov.uk/government/statistics/ndns-results-from-years-7-and-8-combined (Accessed: 8 March 2019).

10 Dendup, T., Feng, X., Clingan, S. and Astell-Burt, T. (2018) 'Environmental Risk Factors for Developing Type 2 Diabetes Mellitus: A Systematic Review.', International journal of environmental research and public health. Multidisciplinary Digital Publishing Institute (MDPI), 15(1). doi: 10.3390/ijerph15010078.

11 Harris, M. L., Oldmeadow, C., Hure, A., Luu, J., Loxton, D. and Attia, J. (2017) 'Stress increases the risk of type 2 diabetes onset in women: A 12-year longitudinal study using causal modelling.', PloS one. Public Library of Science, 12(2), p. e0172126. doi:10.1371/journal.pone.0172126.

12 Taylor, R. and Holman, R. R. (2015) 'Normal weight individuals who develop Type 2 diabetes: the personal fat threshold', Clinical Science, 128(7), pp. 405–410. doi:10.1042/CS20140553.

13 Zhang, N., Yang, X., Zhu, X., Zhao, B., Huang, T. and Ji, Q. (2017) 'Type 2 diabetes mellitus unawareness, prevalence, trends and risk factors: National Health and Nutrition Examination Survey (NHANES) 1999-2010.', The Journal of international medical research. SAGE Publications, 45(2), pp. 594–609. doi: 10.1177/0300060517693178.

14 Jo, A. and Mainous, A. G. (2018) 'Informational value of percent body

fat with body mass index for the risk of abnormal blood glucose: a nationally representative cross-sectional study.', BMJ open. British Medical Journal Publishing Group, 8(4), p. e019200. doi:10.1136/bmjopen-2017-019200.

15 Ma, J., Karlsen, M. C., Chung, M., Jacques, P. F., Saltzman, E., Smith, C. E., Fox, C. S. and McKeown, N. M. (2016) 'Potential link between excess added sugar intake and ectopic fat: a systematic review of randomized controlled trials.', Nutrition reviews. Oxford University Press, 74(1), pp. 18–32. doi: 10.1093/nutrit/nuv047.

16 Maersk, M., Belza, A., Stødkilde-Jørgensen, H., Ringgaard, S., Chabanova, E., Thomsen, H., Pedersen, S. B., Astrup, A. and Richelsen, B. (2012) 'Sucrose-sweetened beverages increase fat storage in the liver, muscle, and visceral fat depot: a 6-mo randomized intervention study', The American Journal of Clinical Nutrition, 95(2), pp. 283–289. doi: 10.3945/ajcn.111.022533.

17 Rippe, J. M. and Angelopoulos, T. J. (2016) 'Relationship between Added Sugars Consumption and Chronic Disease Risk Factors: Current Understanding.', Nutrients. Multidisciplinary Digital Publishing Institute (MDPI), 8(11). doi: 10.3390/nu8110697.

18 Mullie, P., Aerenhouts, D. and Clarys, P. (2012) 'Demographic, socioeconomic and nutritional determinants of daily versus non-daily sugar-sweetened and artificially sweetened beverage consumption', European Journal of Clinical Nutrition, 66(2), pp. 150–155. doi: 10.1038/ejcn.2011.138.

19 van Ansem, W. J. C., van Lenthe, F. J., Schrijvers, C. T. M., Rodenburg, G. and van de Mheen, D. (2014) 'Socio-economic inequalities in children's snack consumption and sugar-sweetened beverage consumption: the contribution of home environmental factors', British Journal of Nutrition, 112(03), pp. 467–476. doi:10.1017/S0007114514001007.

20 DIABETES: FACTS AND STATS (no date). Available at: https://www.diabetes.org.uk/resources-s3/2017-11/diabetes-key-stats-guidelines-april2014.pdf (Accessed: 8 March 2019).

21 Rippe, J. M. and Angelopoulos, T. J. (2016) 'Relationship between Added Sugars Consumption and Chronic Disease Risk Factors: Current Understanding.', Nutrients. Multidisciplinary Digital Publishing Institute (MDPI), 8(11). doi: 10.3390/nu8110697.

22 Macdonald, I. A. (2016) 'A review of recent evidence relating to sugars, insulin resistance and diabetes.', European journal of nutrition. Springer, 55(Suppl 2), pp. 17–23. doi: 10.1007/s00394-016-1340-8.

23 Liberti, M. V and Locasale, J. W. (2016) 'The Warburg Effect: How Does it Benefit Cancer Cells?', Trends in biochemical sciences. NIH Public Access, 41(3), pp. 211–218. doi: 10.1016/j.tibs.2015.12.001.

24 Weber, D. D., Aminazdeh-Gohari, S. and Kofler, B. (2018) 'Ketogenic diet in cancer therapy.', Aging. Impact Journals, LLC, 10(2), pp. 164–165. doi: 10.18632/aging.101382.

25 Rieger, J., Bähr, O., Maurer, G. D., Hattingen, E., Franz, K., Brucker, D., Walenta, S., Kämmerer, U., Coy, J. F., Weller, M. and Steinbach, J. P. (2014) 'Ergo: A pilot study of ketogenic diet in recurrent glioblastoma', International Journal of Oncology, 44(6), pp. 1843–1852. doi: 10.3892/ijo.2014.2382.

26 Martin-McGill, K. J., Srikandarajah, N., Marson, A. G., Tudur Smith, C. and Jenkinson, M. D. (no date) 'The role of ketogenic diets in the therapeutic management of adult and paediatric gliomas: a systematic review'. doi: 10.2217/cns-2017-0030.

27 Weber, D. D., Aminazdeh-Gohari, S. and Kofler, B. (2018) 'Ketogenic diet in cancer therapy.', Aging. Impact Journals, LLC, 10(2), pp. 164–165. doi: 10.18632/aging.101382.

28 Westwater, M. L., Fletcher, P. C. and Ziauddeen, H. (2016) 'Sugar addiction: the state of the science.', European journal of nutrition. Springer, 55(Suppl 2), pp. 55–69. doi:10.1007/s00394-016-1229-6.

29 She's TV's toughest ever weight loss guru, so ... would you spend £1k a week to lose a stone? | Daily Mail Online (no date). Available at: https://www.dailymail.co.uk/news/article-6132119/Shes-TVs-toughest-weight-loss-guru-spend-1k-week-lose-stone.html (Accessed: 8 March 2019).

30 10 signs you're addicted to sugar – and how to detox | Daily Mail Online (no date). Available at: https://www.dailymail.co.uk/health/article-4589584/10-signs-addicted-sugar-detox.html (Accessed: 8 March 2019).

31 Ziauddeen, H., Farooqi, I. S. and Fletcher, P. C. (2012) 'Obesity and the brain: how convincing is the addiction model?', Nature Reviews Neuroscience, 13(4), pp. 279–286. doi: 10.1038/nrn3212.

32 Volkow, N. D. and Wise, R. A. (2005) 'How can drug addiction help us understand obesity?', Nature Neuroscience, 8(5), pp. 555–560. doi: 10.1038/nn1452.

33 Westwater, M. L., Fletcher, P. C. and Ziauddeen, H. (2016) 'Sugar addiction: the state of the science.', European journal of nutrition. Springer, 55(Suppl 2), pp. 55–69. doi:10.1007/s00394-016-1229-6.

34 Wang, G. J., Volkow, N. D., Logan, J., Pappas, N. R., Wong, C. T., Zhu,

W., Netusil, N. and Fowler, J. S. (2001) 'Brain dopamine and obesity.', Lancet (London, England), 357(9253), pp. 354–7. Available at: http://www.ncbi.nlm.nih.gov/pubmed/11210998 (Accessed: 8 March 2019).

35   Long, C. G., Blundell, J. E. and Finlayson, G. (2015) 'A Systematic Review of the Application And Correlates of YFAS-Diagnosed "Food Addiction" in Humans: Are Eating-Related 'Addictions" a Cause for Concern or Empty Concepts?"', Obesity Facts, 8(6), pp. 386–401. doi: 10.1159/000442403.

36   Carter, D. A., Blair, S. E., Cokcetin, N. N., Bouzo, D., Brooks, P., Schothauer, R. and Harry, E. J. (2016) 'Therapeutic Manuka Honey: No Longer So Alternative.', Frontiers in microbiology. Frontiers Media SA, 7, p. 569. doi: 10.3389/fmicb.2016.00569.

37   Geyer, M., Manrique, I., Degen, L. and Beglinger, C. (2008) 'Effect of Yacon (Smallanthus sonchifolius); on Colonic Transit Time in Healthy Volunteers', Digestion, 78(1), pp. 30–33. doi: 10.1159/000155214.

38   Sabater-Molina, M., Larqué, E., Torrella, F. and Zamora, S. (2009) 'Dietary fructooligosaccharides and potential benefits on health', Journal of Physiology and Biochemistry, 65(3), pp. 315–328. doi: 10.1007/BF03180584.

39   Stanhope, K. L., Schwarz, J.-M. and Havel, P. J. (2013) 'Adverse metabolic effects of dietary fructose', Current Opinion in Lipidology, 24(3), pp. 198–206. doi:10.1097/MOL.0b013e3283613bca.

40   Suez, J., Korem, T., Zilberman-Schapira, G., Segal, E. and Elinav, E. (2015) 'Non-caloric artificial sweeteners and the microbiome: findings and challenges', Gut Microbes, 6(2), pp. 149–155. doi: 10.1080/19490976.2015.1017700.

41   Policy Statement – Artificial Sweeteners (no date). Available at: https://www.bda.uk.com/improvinghealth/healthprofessionals/policy_statements/policy_statement_-_artificial_sweeteners (Accessed: 8 March 2019).

42   The truth about sweeteners – NHS (no date). Available at: https://www.nhs.uk/live-well/eat-well/are-sweeteners-safe/ (Accessed: 8 March 2019).

43   'Scientific Opinion on the re-evaluation of aspartame (E 951) as a food additive' (2013) EFSA Journal. John Wiley & Sons, Ltd, 11(12). doi: 10.2903/j.efsa.2013.3496.

44   Policy Statement – Artificial Sweeteners (no date). Available at: https://www.bda.uk.com/improvinghealth/healthprofessionals/policy_statements/policy_statement_-_artificial_sweeteners (Accessed: 8 March 2019).

45 Raben, A. and Richelsen, B. (2012) 'Artificial sweeteners', Current
    Opinion in Clinical Nutrition and Metabolic Care, 15(6), pp. 597–604.
    doi: 10.1097/MCO.0b013e328359678a.

46 Rogers, P. J., Hogenkamp, P. S., de Graaf, C., Higgs, S., Lluch, A.,
    Ness, A. R., Penfold, C., Perry, R., Putz, P., Yeomans, M. R. and Mela,
    D. J. (2016) 'Does low-energy sweetener consumption affect energy
    intake and body weight? A systematic review, including meta-analyses,
    of the evidence from human and animal studies.', International
    journal of obesity (2005). Nature Publishing Group, 40(3), pp. 381–94.
    doi:10.1038/ijo.2015.177.

47 Valdes, A. M., Walter, J., Segal, E. and Spector, T. D. (2018) 'Role of the
    gut microbiota in nutrition and health.', BMJ (Clinical research ed.). British
    Medical Journal Publishing Group, 361, p. k2179. doi: 10.1136/bmj.k2179.

48 Suez, J., Korem, T., Zeevi, D., Zilberman-Schapira, G., Thaiss, C. A.,
    Maza, O., Israeli, D., Zmora, N., Gilad, S., Weinberger, A., Kuperman,
    Y., Harmelin, A., Kolodkin-Gal, I., Shapiro, H., Halpern, Z., Segal, E.
    and Elinav, E. (2014) 'Artificial sweeteners induce glucose intolerance
    by altering the gut microbiota', Nature, 514(7521), pp. 181–186.
    doi:10.1038/nature13793.

49 Suez, J., Korem, T., Zeevi, D., Zilberman-Schapira, G., Thaiss, C. A.,
    Maza, O., Israeli, D., Zmora, N., Gilad, S., Weinberger, A., Kuperman,
    Y., Harmelin, A., Kolodkin-Gal, I., Shapiro, H., Halpern, Z., Segal, E.
    and Elinav, E. (2014) 'Artificial sweeteners induce glucose intolerance
    by altering the gut microbiota', Nature. Nature Publishing Group,
    514(7521), pp. 181–186. doi: 10.1038/nature13793.

50 Suez, J., Korem, T., Zilberman-Schapira, G., Segal, E. and Elinav,
    E. (2015) 'Non-caloric artificial sweeteners and the microbiome:
    findings and challenges', Gut Microbes, 6(2), pp. 149–155. doi:
    10.1080/19490976.2015.1017700.

51 Suez, J., Korem, T., Zilberman-Schapira, G., Segal, E. and Elinav,
    E. (2015) 'Non-caloric artificial sweeteners and the microbiome:
    findings and challenges', Gut Microbes, 6(2), pp. 149–155. doi:
    10.1080/19490976.2015.1017700.

52 Romo-Romo, A., Aguilar-Salinas, C. A., Brito-Córdova, G. X., Gómez
    Díaz, R. A., Vilchis Valentín, D. and Almeda-Valdes, P. (2016) 'Effects
    of the Non-Nutritive Sweeteners on Glucose Metabolism and
    Appetite Regulating Hormones: Systematic Review of Observational
    Prospective Studies and Clinical Trials', PLOS ONE. Edited by C.
    Holscher. Public Library of Science, 11(8), p. e0161264. doi: 10.1371/
    journal.pone.0161264.

53 'Scientific Opinion on the substantiation of health claims related
to intense sweeteners and contribution to the maintenance or
achievement of a normal body weight (ID 1136, 1444, 4299), reduction
of post-prandial glycaemic responses (ID 4298), maintenance' (2011)
EFSA Journal. John Wiley & Sons, Ltd, 9(6), p. 2229. doi:10.2903/j.
efsa.2011.2229.

54 ACNE: British Association of Dermatologists (no date). Available at:
www.bad.org.uk/leaflets (Accessed: 11 March 2019).

55 Fiedler, F., Stangl, G., Fiedler, E. and Taube, K. (2017) 'Acne and
Nutrition: A Systematic Review', Acta Dermato Venereologica, 97(1),
pp. 7–9. doi:10.2340/00015555-2450.

56 Fiedler, F., Stangl, G., Fiedler, E. and Taube, K. (2017) 'Acne and
Nutrition: A Systematic Review', Acta Dermato Venereologica, 97(1),
pp. 7–9. doi: 10.2340/00015555-2450.

Chapter 6 Protein

1 Schoenfeld, B. J., Aragon, A. A. and Krieger, J. W. (2013) 'The effect of
protein timing on muscle strength and hypertrophy: a meta-analysis',
Journal of the International Society of Sports Nutrition, 10(1), p. 53.
doi: 10.1186/1550-2783-10-53.

2 Red Meat and Cancer | How to Prevent Cancer | WCRF UK (no
date). Available at: https://www.wcrf-uk.org/uk/preventing-cancer/
cancer-prevention-recommendations/limit-red-meat-and-avoid-
processed-meat (Accessed: 8 March 2019).

3 Estruch, R., Ros, E., Salas-Salvadó, J., Covas, M.-I., Corella, D., Arós, F.,
Gómez-Gracia, E., Ruiz-Gutiérrez, V., Fiol, M., Lapetra, J., Lamuela-
Raventos, R. M., Serra-Majem, L., Pintó, X., Basora, J., Muñoz, M.
A., Sorlí, J. V., Martínez, J. A., Fitó, M., Gea, A., Hernán, M. A. and
Martínez-González, M. A. (2018) 'Primary Prevention of Cardiovascular
Disease with a Mediterranean Diet Supplemented with Extra-Virgin
Olive Oil or Nuts', New England Journal of Medicine. Massachusetts
Medical Society, 378(25), p. e34. doi: 10.1056/NEJMoa1800389.

4 Rohrmann, S., Overvad, K., Bueno-de-Mesquita, H. B., Jakobsen,
M. U., Egeberg, R., Tjønneland, A., Nailler, L., Boutron-Ruault,
M.-C., Clavel-Chapelon, F., Krogh, V., Palli, D., Panico, S., Tumino,
R., Ricceri, F., Bergmann, M. M., Boeing, H., Li, K., Kaaks, R.,
Khaw, K.-T., Wareham, N. J., Crowe, F. L., Key, T. J., Naska, A.,
Trichopoulou, A., Trichopoulos, D., Leenders, M., Peeters, P. H.,
Engeset, D., Parr, C. L., Skeie, G., Jakszyn, P., Sánchez, M.-J., Huerta,
J. M., Redondo, M. L., Barricarte, A., Amiano, P., Drake, I., Sonestedt,

E., Hallmans, G., Johansson, I., Fedirko, V., Romieux, I., Ferrari, P., Norat, T., Vergnaud, A. C., Riboli, E. and Linseisen, J. (2013) 'Meat consumption and mortality – results from the European Prospective Investigation into Cancer and Nutrition', BMC Medicine, 11(1), p. 63. doi: 10.1186/1741-7015-11-63.

5 Joosen, A. M. C. P., Kuhnle, G. G. C., Aspinall, S. M., Barrow, T. M., Lecommandeur, E., Azqueta, A., Collins, A. R. and Bingham, S. A. (2009) 'Effect of processed and red meat on endogenous nitrosation and DNA damage', Carcinogenesis, 30(8), pp. 1402–1407. doi: 10.1093/carcin/bgp130.

6 Rohrmann, S., Overvad, K., Bueno-de-Mesquita, H. B., Jakobsen, M. U., Egeberg, R., Tjønneland, A., Nailler, L., Boutron-Ruault, M.-C., Clavel-Chapelon, F., Krogh, V., Palli, D., Panico, S., Tumino, R., Ricceri, F., Bergmann, M. M., Boeing, H., Li, K., Kaaks, R., Khaw, K.-T., Wareham, N. J., Crowe, F. L., Key, T. J., Naska, A., Trichopoulou, A., Trichopoulos, D., Leenders, M., Peeters, P. H. M., Engeset, D., Parr, C. L., Skeie, G., Jakszyn, P., Sánchez, M.-J., Huerta, J. M., Redondo, M. L., Barricarte, A., Amiano, P., Drake, I., Sonestedt, E., Hallmans, G., Johansson, I., Fedirko, V., Romieux, I., Ferrari, P., Norat, T., Vergnaud, A. C., Riboli, E. and Linseisen, J. (2013) 'Meat consumption and mortality--results from the European Prospective Investigation into Cancer and Nutrition.', BMC medicine. BioMed Central, 11, p. 63. doi: 10.1186/1741-7015-11-63.

7 Processed meat and cancer – what you need to know – Cancer Research UK – Science blog (no date). Available at: https://scienceblog.cancerresearchuk.org/2015/10/26/processed-meat-and-cancer-whatyou-need-to-know/ (Accessed: 8 March 2019).

8 Van Elswyk, M. E., Weatherford, C. A. and McNeill, S. H. (2018) 'A Systematic Review of Renal Health in Healthy Individuals Associated with Protein Intake above the US Recommended Daily Allowance in Randomized Controlled Trials and Observational Studies', Advances in Nutrition. Oxford University Press, 9(4), pp. 404–418. doi:10.1093/advances/nmy026.

9 Kamper, A.-L. and Strandgaard, S. (2017) 'Long-Term Effects of High-Protein Diets on Renal Function', Annual Review of Nutrition. Annual Reviews, 37(1), pp. 347–369. doi:10.1146/annurev-nutr-071714-034426.

10 Haring, B., Selvin, E., Liang, M., Coresh, J., Grams, M. E., Petruski-Ivleva, N., Steffen, L. M. and Rebholz, C. M. (2017) 'Dietary Protein Sources and Risk for Incident Chronic Kidney Disease: Results From the Atherosclerosis Risk in Communities (ARIC) Study.', Journal of

renal nutrition : the official journal of the Council on Renal Nutrition of the National Kidney Foundation. Elsevier, 27(4), pp. 233–242. doi:10.1053/j.jrn.2016.11.004.

11 Van Elswyk, M. E., Weatherford, C. A. and McNeill, S. H. (2018) 'A Systematic Review of Renal Health in Healthy Individuals Associated with Protein Intake above the US Recommended Daily Allowance in Randomized Controlled Trials and Observational Studies', Advances in Nutrition, 9(4), pp. 404–418. doi: 10.1093/advances/nmy026.

12 Murphy, C. H., Hector, A. J. and Phillips, S. M. (2015) 'Considerations for protein intake in managing weight loss in athletes', European Journal of Sport Science. Routledge, 15(1), pp. 21–28. doi: 10.1080/17461391.2014.936325.

13 Simmons, E., Fluckey, J. D. and Riechman, S. E. (2016) 'Cumulative Muscle Protein Synthesis and Protein Intake Requirements', Annual Review of Nutrition. Annual Reviews , 36(1), pp. 17–43. doi: 10.1146/annurev-nutr-071813-105549.

14 NDNS: results from years 7 and 8 (combined) – GOV.UK (no date). Available at: https://www.gov.uk/government/statistics/ndns-results-from-years-7-and-8-combined (Accessed: 8 March 2019).

Chapter 7 Micronutrients and Supplements

1 Carpenter, K. J. (2012) 'The Discovery of Vitamin C', Annals of Nutrition and Metabolism, 61(3), pp. 259–264. doi: 10.1159/000343121.

2 Semba, R. D. (2012) 'The Discovery of the Vitamins', International Journal for Vitamin and Nutrition Research, 82(5), pp. 310–315. doi: 10.1024/0300-9831/a000124.

3 Global Dietary Supplements Market Size & Trends Analysis, 2016 to 2022 (no date). Available at: https://www.zionmarketresearch.com/report/dietary-supplements-market (Accessed: 8 March 2019).

4 Industry Facts – Health Food Manufacturers' Association (no date). Available at: https://www.hfma.co.uk/media-events/industry-facts/ (Accessed: 8 March 2019).

5 Fortmann, S. P., Burda, B. U., Senger, C. A., Lin, J. S. and Whitlock, E. P. (2013) 'Vitamin and Mineral Supplements in the Primary Prevention of Cardiovascular Disease and Cancer: An Updated Systematic Evidence Review for the U.S. Preventive ServicesTask Force', Annals of Internal Medicine. American College of Physicians, 159(12), pp. 824–834. doi: 10.7326/0003-4819-159-12-201312170-00729.

6 Bjelakovic, G., Nikolova, D., Gluud, L. L., Simonetti, R. G. and Gluud, C. (2012) 'Antioxidant supplements for prevention of mortality

in healthy participants and patients with various diseases', Cochrane Database of Systematic Reviews. doi:10.1002/14651858.CD007176. pub2.

Chapter 9 Balanced Eating

1 Lobo, V., Patil, A., Phatak, A. and Chandra, N. (2010) 'Free radicals, antioxidants and functional foods: Impact on human health.', Pharmacognosy reviews. Wolters Kluwer–Medknow Publications, 4(8), pp. 118–26. doi: 10.4103/0973-7847.70902.

2 Hodges, R. E. and Minich, D. M. (2015) 'Modulation of Metabolic Detoxification Pathways Using Foods and Food-Derived Components: A Scientific Review with Clinical Application.', Journal of nutrition and metabolism. Hindawi Limited, 2015, p. 760689. doi:10.1155/2015/760689.

3 Liu, R. H. (2013) 'Health-promoting components of fruits and vegetables in the diet.', Advances in nutrition (Bethesda, Md.). American Society for Nutrition, 4(3), p. 384S–92S. doi: 10.3945/an.112.003517.

4 Bouzari, A., Holstege, D. and Barrett, D. M. (2015) 'Vitamin Retention in Eight Fruits and Vegetables: A Comparison of Refrigerated and Frozen Storage', Journal of Agricultural and Food Chemistry, 63(3), pp. 957–962. doi: 10.1021/jf5058793.

5 Bedford, J. L. and Barr, S. I. (2005) 'Diets and selected lifestyle practices of self-defined adult vegetarians from a population-based sample suggest they are more "health conscious"', International Journal of Behavioral Nutrition and Physical Activity, 2(1), p. 4. doi: 10.1186/1479-5868-2-4.

6 Satija, A., Bhupathiraju, S. N., Spiegelman, D., Chiuve, S. E., Manson, J. E., Willett, W., Rexrode, K. M., Rimm, E. B. and Hu, F. B. (2017) 'Healthful and Unhealthful Plant-Based Diets and the Risk of Coronary Heart Disease in U.S. Adults', Journal of the American College of Cardiology. Journal of the American College of Cardiology, 70(4), pp. 411–422. doi: 10.1016/j.jacc.2017.05.047.

7 Dinu, M., Abbate, R., Gensini, G. F., Casini, A. and Sofi, F. (2017) 'Vegetarian, vegan diets and multiple health outcomes: A systematic review with meta-analysis of observational studies', Critical Reviews in Food Science and Nutrition, 57(17), pp. 3640–3649. doi: 10.1080/10408398.2016.1138447.

8 Wright, N., Wilson, L., Smith, M., Duncan, B. and Mchugh, P. (2017) 'The BROAD study: A randomised controlled trial using a whole food

plant-based diet in the community for obesity, ischaemic heart disease or diabetes', Nutrition & Diabetes, 7, p. 256. doi:10.1038/nutd.2017.3.

9   Martínez-González, M. A., Salas-Salvadó, J., Estruch, R., Corella, D., Fitó, M., Ros, E. and PREDIMED INVESTIGATORS (2015) 'Benefits of the Mediterranean Diet: Insights From the PREDIMED Study', Progress in Cardiovascular Diseases, 58(1), pp. 50–60. doi: 10.1016/j.pcad.2015.04Berild, A., Holven, K. B. and Ulven, S. M. (2017) 'Anbefalt nordisk kosthold og risikomarkører for hjerte- og karsykdom', Tidsskrift for Den norske legeforening, 137(10), pp. 721–726. doi: 10.4045/tidsskr.16.0243..003.

10 Berild, A., Holven, K. B. and Ulven, S. M. (2017) 'Anbefalt nordisk kosthold og risikomarkører for hjerte – og karsykdom', Tidsskrift for Den norske legeforening, 137(10), pp. 721–726. doi: 10.4045/tidsskr.16.0243.

11 Key, T. J., Appleby, P. N., Spencer, E. A., Travis, R. C., Roddam, A. W. and Allen, N. E. (2009) 'Cancer incidence in vegetarians: results from the European Prospective Investigation into Cancer and Nutrition (EPIC-Oxford)', The American Journal of Clinical Nutrition. Oxford University Press, 89(5), p. 1620S–1626S. doi:10.3945/ajcn.2009.26736M.

12 Spence, J. D., Jenkins, D. J. A. and Davignon, J. (2012) 'Egg yolk consumption and carotid plaque', Atherosclerosis. Elsevier, 224(2), pp. 469–473. doi:10.1016/J.ATHEROSCLEROSIS.2012.07.032.

13 Bonjour, J.-P. (2013) 'Nutritional disturbance in acid–base balance and osteoporosis: a hypothesis that disregards the essential homeostatic role of the kidney', British Journal of Nutrition, 110(07), pp. 1168–1177. doi: 10.1017/S0007114513000962

14 Rizzoli, R., Biver, E., Bonjour, J.-P., Coxam, V., Goltzman, D., Kanis, J. A., Lappe, J., Rejnmark, L., Sahni, S., Weaver, C., Weiler, H. and Reginster, J.-Y. (2018) 'Benefits and safety of dietary protein for bone health—an expert consensus paper endorsed by the European Society for Clinical and Economical Aspects of Osteopororosis, Osteoarthritis, and Musculoskeletal Diseases and by the International Osteoporosis Foundation', Osteoporosis International, 29(9), pp. 1933–1948. doi: 10.1007/s00198-018-4534-5.

15 van den Heuvel, E. G. H. M. and Steijns, J. M. J. M. (2018) 'Dairy products and bone health: how strong is the scientific evidence?', Nutrition Research Reviews, 31(2), pp. 164–178. doi: 10.1017/S095442241800001X.

16 Bonjour, J.-P. (2013) 'Nutritional disturbance in acid–base balance and osteoporosis: a hypothesis that disregards the essential homeostatic role of the kidney', British Journal of Nutrition, 110(07), pp. 1168–1177. doi: 10.1017/S0007114513000962.

17 Study of Current and Former Vegetarians and Vegans Secondary Findings (2016). Available at: https://faunalytics.org/wp-content/uploads/2016/02/Faunalytics-Study-of-Current-and-Former-Vegetarians-and-Vegans---Secondary-Findings-.pdf (Accessed: 11 March 2019).

18 Lietz, G., Oxley, A., Leung, W. and Hesketh, J. (2012) 'Single Nucleotide Polymorphisms Upstream from the β-Carotene 15,15'-Monoxygenase Gene Influence Provitamin A Conversion Efficiency in Female Volunteers', The Journal of Nutrition, 142(1), p. 161S–165S. doi: 10.3945/jn.111.140756.

19 Karl, J. P., Fu, X., Wang, X., Zhao, Y., Shen, J., Zhang, C., Wolfe, B. E., Saltzman, E., Zhao, L. and Booth, S. L. (2015) 'Fecal menaquinone profiles of overweight adults are associated with gut microbiota composition during a gut microbiota–targeted dietary intervention', The American Journal of Clinical Nutrition, 102(1), pp. 84–93. doi:10.3945/ajcn.115.109496.

20 What is a sustainable healthy diet? A discussion paper | CCAFS: CGIAR research program on Climate Change, Agriculture and Food Security (no date). Available at: https://ccafs.cgiar.org/publications/what-sustainable-healthy-diet-discussion-paper#.XIPhlq2caCR (Accessed: 9 March 2019).

21 Aleksandrowicz, L., Green, R., Joy, E. J. M., Smith, P. and Haines, A. (2016) 'The Impacts of Dietary Change on Greenhouse Gas Emissions, Land Use, Water Use, and Health: A Systematic Review', PLOS ONE. Edited by A. S. Wiley. Public Library of Science, 11(11), p. e0165797. doi: 10.1371/journal.pone.0165797.

22 Rosi, A., Mena, P., Pellegrini, N., Turroni, S., Neviani, E., Ferrocino, I., Di Cagno, R., Ruini, L., Ciati, R., Angelino, D., Maddock, J., Gobbetti, M., Brighenti, F., Del Rio, D. and Scazzina, F. (2017) 'Environmental impact of omnivorous, ovo-lacto-vegetarian, and vegan diet', Scientific Reports, 7(1), p. 6105. doi: 10.1038/s41598-017-06466-8.

23 Aleksandrowicz, L., Green, R., Joy, E. J. M., Smith, P. and Haines, A. (2016) 'The Impacts of Dietary Change on Greenhouse Gas Emissions, Land Use, Water Use, and Health: A Systematic Review', PLOS ONE. Edited by A. S. Wiley, 11(11), p. e0165797.doi: 10.1371/journal.pone.0165797.

Chapter 10 Eating for a Healthy Gut

1 Bianconi, E., Piovesan, A., Facchin, F., Beraudi, A., Casadei, R., Frabetti, F., Vitale, L., Pelleri, M. C., Tassani, S., Piva, F., Perez-Amodio, S., Strippoli, P. and Canaider, S. (2013) 'An estimation of the number of cells

in the human body', Annals of Human Biology, 40(6), pp. 463–471. doi: 10.3109/03014460.2013.807878.

2 Clapp, M., Aurora, N., Herrera, L., Bhatia, M., Wilen, E. and Wakefield, S. (2017) 'Gut microbiota's effect on mental health: The gut-brain axis.', Clinics and practice. PAGEPress, 7(4), p. 987. doi: 10.4081/cp.2017.987.

3 Vandenplas, Y., Zakharova, I. and Dmitrieva, Y. (2015) 'Oligosaccharides in infant formula: more evidence to validate the role of prebiotics', British Journal of Nutrition, 113(09), pp. 1339 1344. doi: 10.1017/S0007114515000823.

4 Valdes, A. M., Walter, J., Segal, E. and Spector, T. D. (2018) 'Role of the gut microbiota in nutrition and health.', BMJ (Clinical research ed.). British Medical Journal Publishing Group, 361, p. k2179. doi: 10.1136/bmj.k2179.

5 Sanders, M. E., Merenstein, D., Merrifield, C. A. and Hutkins, R. (2018) 'Probiotics for human use', Nutrition Bulletin. John Wiley & Sons, Ltd (10.1111), 43(3), pp. 212–225. doi: 10.1111/nbu.12334.

6 Richards, D. G., McMillin, D. L., Mein, E. A. and Nelson, C. D. (2006) 'Colonic Irrigations: A Review of the Historical Controversy and the Potential for Adverse Effects', The Journal of Alternative and Complementary Medicine, 12(4), pp. 389–393. doi:10.1089/acm.2006.12.389.

7 Mishori R, et al. (no date) The dangers of colon cleansing. Available at: https://www.mdedge.com/sites/default/files/Document/September-2017/6008JFP_Article1.pdf (Accessed: 9 March 2019).

8 Dore, M. and Gleeson, T. (2015) 'Escherichia coli Septic Shock Following Colonic Hydrotherapy', The American Journal of Medicine, 128(10), p. e31. doi:10.1016/j.amjmed.2015.05.032.

9 Cummings, J. H., Antoine, J.-M., Azpiroz, F., Bourdet-Sicard, R., Brandtzaeg, P., Calder, P. C., Gibson, G. R., Guarner, F., Isolauri, E., Pannemans, D., Shortt, C., Tuijtelaars, S. and Watzl, B. (2004) 'PASSCLAIM1?Gut health and immunity', European Journal of Nutrition, 43(S2), pp. ii118–ii173. doi: 10.1007/s00394-004-1205-4.

10 sacn (2015) Carbohydrates and Health. Available at: www.tsoshop.co.uk (Accessed: 10 March 2019).

11 Burkitt, D. P., Walker, A. R. and Painter, N. S. (1972) 'Effect of dietary fibre on stools and the transit-times, and its role in the causation of disease.', Lancet (London, England), 2(7792), pp. 1408–12. Available at: http://www.ncbi.nlm.nih.gov/pubmed/4118696 (Accessed: 10 March 2019).

12   Mohajeri, M. H., La Fata, G., Steinert, R. E. and Weber, P. (2018) 'Relationship between the gut microbiome and brain function', Nutrition Reviews, 76(7), pp. 481–496. doi:10.1093/nutrit/nuy009.

13   Ng, Q. X., Peters, C., Ho, C. Y. X., Lim, D. Y. and Yeo, W.-S. (2018) 'A meta-analysis of the use of probiotics to alleviate depressive symptoms', Journal of Affective Disorders, 228, pp. 13–19. doi: 10.1016/j.jad.2017.11.063.

14   Williams, J. G., Roberts, S. E., Ali, M. F., Cheung, W. Y., Cohen, D. R., Demery, G., Edwards, A., Greer, M., Hellier, M. D., Hutchings, H. A., Ip, B., Longo, M. F., Russell, I. T., Snooks, H. A. and Williams, J. C. (2007) 'Gastroenterology services in the UK. The burden of disease, and the organisation and delivery of services for gastrointestinal and liver disorders: a review of the evidence.', Gut. BMJ Publishing Group, 56 Suppl 1(Suppl1), pp. 1–113. doi: 10.1136/gut.2006.117598.

15   Common digestive problems – and how to treat them – NHS (no date). Available at: https://www.nhs.uk/live-well/eat-well/common-digestive-problems-and-how-to-treat-them/ (Accessed: 10 March 2019).

16   McKenzie, Y. A., Bowyer, R. K., Leach, H., Gulia, P., Horobin, J., O'Sullivan, N. A., Pettitt, C., Reeves, L. B., Seamark, L., Williams, M., Thompson, J., Lomer, M. C. E. and (IBS Dietetic Guideline Review Group on behalf of Gastroenterology Specialist Group of the British Dietetic Association) (2016) 'British Dietetic Association systematic review and evidence-based practice guidelines for the dietary management of irritable bowel syndrome in adults (2016 update)', Journal of Human Nutrition and Dietetics, 29(5), pp. 549–575. doi: 10.1111/jhn.12385.

17   Staudacher, H. M. and Whelan, K. (2017) 'The low FODMAP diet: recent advances in understanding its mechanisms and efficacy in IBS', Gut, 66(8), pp. 1517–1527. doi:10.1136/gutjnl-2017-313750.

18   McKenzie, Y. A., Bowyer, R. K., Leach, H., Gulia, P., Horobin, J., O'Sullivan, N. A., Pettitt, C., Reeves, L. B., Seamark, L., Williams, M., Thompson, J., Lomer, M. C. E. and (IBS Dietetic Guideline Review Group on behalf of Gastroenterology Specialist Group of the British Dietetic Association) (2016) 'British Dietetic Association systematic review and evidence-based practice guidelines for the dietary management of irritable bowel syndrome in adults (2016 update)', Journal of Human Nutrition and Dietetics, 29(5), pp. 549–575. doi: 10.1111/jhn.12385.

19   Qin, H.-Y., Cheng, C.-W., Tang, X.-D. and Bian, Z.-X. (2014) 'Impact of psychological stress on irritable bowel syndrome.', World journal

of gastroenterology. Baishideng Publishing Group Inc, 20(39), pp. 14126–31. doi: 10.3748/wjg.v20.i39.14126.

20 'Overview | Irritable bowel syndrome in adults: diagnosis and management | Guidance | NICE' (no date). NICE. Available at: https:// www.nice.org.uk/guidance/cg61 (Accessed: 9 March 2019).

21 Gibson, P. R. (2017) 'History of the low FODMAP diet', Journal of Gastroenterology and Hepatology, 32, pp. 5–7. doi: 10.1111/jgh.13685.

22 O'Keeffe, M., Jansen, C., Martin, L., Williams, M., Seamark, L., Staudacher, H. M., Irving, P. M., Whelan, K. and Lomer, M. C. (2018) 'Long-term impact of the low-FODMAP diet on gastrointestinal symptoms, dietary intake, patient acceptability, and healthcare utilization in irritable bowel syndrome', Neurogastroenterology & Motility. John Wiley & Sons, Ltd (10.1111), 30(1), p. e13154. doi: 10.1111/ nmo.13154.

23 Staudacher, H. M. and Whelan, K. (2017) 'The low FODMAP diet: recent advances in understanding its mechanisms and efficacy in IBS', Gut, 66(8), pp. 1517–1527. doi:10.1136/gutjnl-2017-313750.

24 Altobelli, E., Del Negro, V., Angeletti, P. and Latella, G. (2017) 'Low-FODMAP Diet Improves Irritable Bowel Syndrome Symptoms: A Meta-Analysis', Nutrients, 9(9), p. 940. doi: 10.3390/nu9090940.

25 Halmos, E. P., Christophersen, C. T., Bird, A. R., Shepherd, S. J., Gibson, P. R. and Muir, J. G. (2015) 'Diets that differ in their FODMAP content alter the colonic luminal microenvironment', Gut, 64(1), pp. 93–100. doi: 10.1136/gutjnl-2014-307264.

26 Jalanka-Tuovinen, J., Salonen, A., Nikkilä, J., Immonen, O., Kekkonen, R., Lahti, L., Palva, A. and de Vos, W. M. (2011) 'Intestinal Microbiota in Healthy Adults: Temporal Analysis Reveals Individual and Common Core and Relation to Intestinal Symptoms', PLoS ONE. Edited by S. Bereswill. Public Library of Science, 6(7), p. e23035. doi:10.1371/ journal.pone.0023035.

27 O'Keeffe, M., Jansen, C., Martin, L., Williams, M., Seamark, L., Staudacher, H. M., Irving, P. M., Whelan, K. and Lomer, M. C. (2018) 'Long-term impact of the low-FODMAP diet on gastrointestinal symptoms, dietary intake, patient acceptability, and healthcare utilization in irritable bowel syndrome', Neurogastroenterology & Motility. John Wiley & Sons, Ltd (10.1111), 30(1), p. e13154. doi: 10.1111/nmo.13154.

28 Harper, A., Naghibi, M., Garcha, D., Harper, A., Naghibi, M. M. and Garcha, D. (2018) 'The Role of Bacteria, Probiotics and Diet in Irritable Bowel Syndrome', Foods. Multidisciplinary Digital Publishing Institute, 7(2), p. 13. doi: 10.3390/foods7020013.

29   Healey, G. R., Murphy, R., Brough, L., Butts, C. A. and Coad, J. (2017)
     'Interindividual variability in gut microbiota and host response to
     dietary interventions', Nutrition Reviews. Oxford University Press,
     75(12), pp. 1059–1080. doi: 10.1093/nutrit/nux062.

Chapter 11 Eating with Allergies and Intolerances

1   Tang, M. L. K. and Mullins, R. J. (2017) 'Food allergy: is prevalence
    increasing?', Internal Medicine Journal, 47(3), pp. 256–261. doi: 10.1111/
    imj.13362.

2   Tang, M. L. K. and Mullins, R. J. (2017) 'Food allergy: is prevalence
    increasing?', Internal Medicine Journal, 47(3), pp. 256–261. doi: 10.1111/
    imj.13362.

3   Turner, P. J., Gowland, M. H., Sharma, V., Ierodiakonou, D., Harper,
    N., Garcez, T., Pumphrey, R. and Boyle, R. J. (2015) 'Increase in
    anaphylaxis-related hospitalizations but no increase in fatalities: an
    analysis of United Kingdom national anaphylaxis data, 1992-2012.', The
    Journal of allergy and clinical immunology. Elsevier, 135(4), p. 956–63.
    e1. doi: 10.1016/j.jaci.2014.10.021.

4   Nwaru, B. I., Hickstein, L., Panesar, S. S., Roberts, G., Muraro, A. and
    Sheikh, A. (2014) 'Prevalence of common food allergies in Europe: a
    systematic review and meta-analysis', Allergy. John Wiley & Sons, Ltd
    (10.1111), 69(8), pp. 992–1007. doi:10.1111/all.12423.

5   Okada, H., Kuhn, C., Feillet, H. and Bach, J.-F. (2010) 'The "hygiene
    hypothesis" for autoimmune and allergic diseases: an update.', Clinical
    and experimental immunology. Wiley-Blackwell, 160(1), pp. 1–9. doi:
    10.1111/j.1365-2249.2010.04139.x.

6   Venter, C., Brown, T., Meyer, R., Walsh, J., Shah, N., Nowak-
    We.grzyn, A., Chen, T.-X., Fleischer, D. M., Heine, R. G., Levin,
    M., Vieira, M. C. and Fox, A. T. (2017) 'Better recognition, diagnosis
    and management of non-IgE-mediated cow's milk allergy in infancy:
    iMAP—an international interpretation of the MAP (Milk Allergy in
    Primary Care) guideline', Clinical and Translational Allergy. BioMed
    Central, 7(1), p. 26. doi:10.1186/s13601-017-0162-y.

7   Molina-Infante, J., Santolaria, S., Sanders, D. S. and Fernández-
    Bañares, F. (2015) 'Systematic review: noncoeliac gluten sensitivity',
    Alimentary Pharmacology & Therapeutics, 41(9), pp. 807–820. doi:
    10.1111/apt.13155.

8   Ellis, A. and Linaker, B. D. (1978) 'Non-coeliac gluten sensitivity?',
    Lancet (London, England), 1(8078), pp. 1358–9. Available at: http://
    www.ncbi.nlm.nih.gov/pubmed/78118 (Accessed: 9 March 2019).

9   Skodje, G. I., Sarna, V. K., Minelle, I. H., Rolfsen, K. L., Muir, J. G., Gibson, P. R., Veierød, M. B., Henriksen, C. and Lundin, K. E. A. (2018) 'Fructan, Rather Than Gluten, Induces Symptoms in Patients With Self-Reported Non-Celiac Gluten Sensitivity', Gastroenterology, 154(3), p. 529–539.e2. doi: 10.1053/j.gastro.2017.10.040.

10 Molina-Infante, J., Santolaria, S., Sanders, D. S. and Fernández-Bañares, F. (2015) 'Systematic review: noncoeliac gluten sensitivity', Alimentary Pharmacology & Therapeutics, 41(9), pp. 807–820. doi: 10.1111/apt.13155.

11 Biesiekierski, J. R. and Iven, J. (2015) 'Non coeliac gluten sensitivity: piecing the puzzle together.', United European gastroenterology journal. SAGE Publications, 3(2), pp. 160–5. doi: 10.1177/2050640615578388.

12 Gocki, J. and Bartuzi, Z. (2016) 'Role of immunoglobulin G antibodies in diagnosis of food allergy.', Postepy dermatologii i alergologii. Termedia Publishing, 33(4), pp. 253–6. doi: 10.5114/ada.2016.61600.

13 Carr, S., Chan, E., Lavine, E. and Moote, W. (2012) 'CSACI Position statement on the testing of food-specific IgG.', Allergy, asthma, and clinical immunology : official journal of the Canadian Society of Allergy and Clinical Immunology. BioMed Central, 8(1), p. 12. doi: 10.1186/1710-1492-8-12.

14 Katelaris, C. H., Weiner, J. M., Heddle, R. J., Stuckey, M. S. and Yan, K. W. (1991) 'Vega testing in the diagnosis of allergic conditions. The Australian College of Allergy.', The Medical journal of Australia, 155(2), pp. 113–4. Available at: http://www.ncbi.nlm.nih.gov/pubmed/1857287 (Accessed: 9 March 2019).

15 Austin, M. and Bloomfield, S. (no date) HETAL DHRUVE Barts Heath NHS Trust. Available at: www.senseaboutscience.org/pages/ (Accessed: 9 March 2019).

Chapter 12 Diet Culture and Weight Stigma

1   Party Parliamentary Group on Body Image, A. (2011) Reflections on body image. Available at: http://ymca-central-assets.s3-eu-west-1.amazonaws.com/s3fs-public/APPG-Reflectionson-body-image.pdf (Accessed: 9 March 2019).

2   Body Confidence Progress Report 2015 – GOV.UK (no date). Available at: https://www.gov.uk/government/publications/body-confidence-progress-report-2015 (Accessed: 9 March 2019).

3   BBC Radio 5 Live – Plastic Surgery and Cosmetic Procedures « ComRes (no date). Available at: https://www.comresglobal.com/polls/bbc-radio-5-live-plastic-surgery-and-cosmetic-procedures/ (Accessed: 9 March 2019).

4   Steroids see four-fold increase, data shows, fuelled by rise in muscle-conscious young men (no date). Available at: https://www.telegraph.co.uk/news/2017/07/27/steroids-see-four-fold-increase-data-shows-fuelled-rise-muscle/ (Accessed: 9 March 2019).

5   #fitspo Instagram images. Available at: https://www.instagram.com/explore/tags/fitspo/?hl=en (Accessed: 9 March 2019).

6   Boepple, L. and Thompson, J. K. (2016) 'A content analytic comparison of fitspiration and thinspiration websites', International Journal of Eating Disorders, 49(1), pp. 98–101. doi: 10.1002/eat.22403.

7   Sharpe, H., Griffiths, S., Choo, T., Eisenberg, M. E., Mitchison, D., Wall, M. and Neumark-Sztainer, D. (2018) 'The relative importance of dissatisfaction, overvaluation and preoccupation with weight and shape for predicting onset of disordered eating behaviors and depressive symptoms over 15 years', International Journal of Eating Disorders, 51(10), pp. 1168–1175. doi: 10.1002/eat.22936.

8   Vartanian, L. R. and Porter, A. M. (2016) 'Weight stigma and eating behavior: A review of the literature', Appetite, 102, pp. 3–14. doi: 10.1016/j.appet.2016.01.034.

9   Neumark-Sztainer, D., Falkner, N., Story, M., Perry, C., Hannan, P. and Mulert, S. (2002) 'Weight-teasing among adolescents: correlations with weight status and disordered eating behaviors', International Journal of Obesity, 26(1), pp. 123–131. doi:10.1038/sj.ijo.0801853.

10 Mulgrew, K. E., McCulloch, K., Farren, E., Prichard, I. and Lim, M. S. C. (2018) 'This girl can #jointhemovement: Effectiveness of physical functionality-focused campaigns for women's body satisfaction and exercise intent', Body Image, 24, pp. 26–35. doi:10.1016/j.bodyim.2017.11.007.

11 Nutter, S., Russell-Mayhew, S., Alberga, A. S., Arthur, N., Kassan, A., Lund, D. E., Sesma-Vazquez, M. and Williams, E. (2016) 'Positioning of Weight Bias: Moving towards Social Justice.', Journal of obesity. Hindawi Limited, 2016, p. 3753650. doi:10.1155/2016/3753650.

12 Puhl, R. M. and Heuer, C. A. (2010) 'Obesity stigma: important considerations for public health.', American journal of public health. American Public Health Association, 100(6), pp. 1019–28. doi: 10.2105/AJPH.2009.159491.

13 Swift, J. A., Hanlon, S., El-Redy, L., Puhl, R. M. and Glazebrook, C. (2013) 'Weight bias among UK trainee dietitians, doctors, nurses and nutritionists', Journal of Human Nutrition and Dietetics, 26(4), pp. 395–402. doi: 10.1111/jhn.12019.

14 Foster, G. D., Wadden, T. A., Makris, A. P., Davidson, D., Sanderson,

R. S., Allison, D. B. and Kessler, A. (2003) 'Primary Care Physicians' Attitudes about Obesity and Its Treatment', Obesity Research, 11(10), pp. 1168–1177. doi: 10.1038/oby.2003.161.

15 Puhl, R. M. and Heuer, C. A. (2010) 'Obesity stigma: important considerations for public health.', American journal of public health. American Public Health Association, 100(6), pp. 1019–28. doi: 10.2105/ AJPH.2009.159491./

16 Wu, Y.-K. and Berry, D. C. (2018) 'Impact of weight stigma on physiological and psychological health outcomes for overweight and obese adults: A systematic review', Journal of Advanced Nursing, 74(5), pp. 1030–1042. doi: 10.1111/jan.13511.

17 Phelan, S. M., Burgess, D. J., Yeazel, M. W., Hellerstedt, W. L., Griffin, J. M. and van Ryn, M. (2015) 'Impact of weight bias and stigma on quality of care and outcomes for patients with obesity.', Obesity reviews : an official journal of the International Association for the Study of Obesity. Wiley-Blackwell, 16(4), pp. 319–26. doi:10.1111/ obr.12266.

18 Swift, J. A., Hanlon, S., El-Redy, L., Puhl, R. M. and Glazebrook, C. (2013) 'Weight bias among UK trainee dietitians, doctors, nurses and nutritionists', Journal of Human Nutrition and Dietetics, 26(4), pp. 395–402. doi: 10.1111/jhn.12019.

19 Tomiyama, A. J., Carr, D., Granberg, E. M., Major, B., Robinson, E., Sutin, A. R. and Brewis, A. (2018) 'How and why weight stigma drives the obesity "epidemic" and harms health.', BMC medicine. BioMed Central, 16(1), p. 123. doi: 10.1186/s12916-018-1116-5.

20 Puhl, R. and Suh, Y. (2015) 'Health Consequences of Weight Stigma: Implications for Obesity Prevention and Treatment', Current Obesity Reports, 4(2), pp. 182–190. doi:10.1007.

21 Schaefer, J. T. and Magnuson, A. B. (2014) 'A Review of Interventions that Promote Eating by Internal Cues', *Journal of the Academy of Nutrition and Dietetics* . Elsevier, 114(5), pp. 734–760. doi: 10.1016/J. JAND.2013.12.024.

22 Schaefer, J. T. and Magnuson, A. B. (2014) 'A Review of Interventions that Promote Eating by Internal Cues', Journal of the Academy of Nutrition and Dietetics. Elsevier, 114(5), pp. 734–760. doi: 10.1016/J. JAND.2013.12.024.

23 Van Dyke, N. and Drinkwater, E. J. (2014) 'Review Article Relationships between intuitive eating and health indicators: literature review', *Public Health Nutrition* , 17(08), pp. 1757–1766. doi: 10.1017/ S1368980013002139.

24 Van Dyke, N. and Drinkwater, E. J. (2014) 'Review Article Relationships between intuitive eating and health indicators: literature review', Public Health Nutrition, 17(08), pp. 1757–1766. doi: 10.1017/S1368980013002139.

Chapter 13 Popular Diets and Nutrition

1 Victoria Beckham reveals Alkaline diet as secret to her super slimline figure – Daily Record (no date). Available at: https://www.dailyrecord.co.uk/entertainment/celebrity/victoria-beckham-reveals-alkalinediet-1530648 (Accessed: 9 March 2019).

2 Elle Macpherson talks to Dr Simoné, her personal nutritionist, from Rejuv. | Rejuv (no date). Available at: http://www.rejuv.co.uk/blog/elle-macpherson-talks-about-the-super-elixir-with-dr-simone-laubscher (Accessed: 9 March 2019).

3 Robet O. Young – Wikipedia. Available at: https://en.wikipedia.org/wiki/Robert_O._Young . (Accessed: 9 March 2019).

4 Fenton, T. R. and Huang, T. (2016) 'Systematic review of the association between dietary acid load, alkaline water and cancer.', BMJ open. BMJ Publishing Group, 6(6), p. e010438. doi: 10.1136/bmjopen-2015-010438.

5 Schwalfenberg, G. K. (2012) 'The alkaline diet: is there evidence that an alkaline pH diet benefits health?', Journal of environmental and public health. Hindawi Limited, 2012, p. 727630. doi: 10.1155/2012/727630.

6 Robey, I. F. (2012) 'Examining the relationship between diet-induced acidosis and cancer', Nutrition & Metabolism. BioMed Central, 9(1), p. 72. doi:10.1186/1743-7075-9-72.

7 Fenton, T. R., Tough, S. C., Lyon, A. W., Eliasziw, M. and Hanley, D. A. (2011) 'Causal assessment of dietary acid load and bone disease: a systematic review &meta-analysis applying Hill's epidemiologic criteria for causality.', Nutrition journal. BioMed Central, 10, p. 41. doi: 10.1186/1475-2891-10-41.

8 Han, E., Kim, G., Hong, N., Lee, Y.-H., Kim, D. W., Shin, H. J., Lee, B.-W., Kang, E. S., Lee, I.-K. and Cha, B.-S. (2016) 'Association between dietary acid load and the risk of cardiovascular disease: nationwide surveys (KNHANES 2008-2011).', Cardiovascular diabetology. BioMed Central, 15(1), p. 122. doi: 10.1186/s12933-016-0436-z.

9 My beef with Jordan Peterson's all-cow diet | Emer O"Toole | Opinion | The Guardian (no date). Available at: https://www.theguardian.com/

commentisfree/2018/sep/19/my-beef-with-jordan-petersons-all-cow-diet (Accessed: 9 March 2019).

10 They mock vegans and eat 4lb of steak a day: meet 'carnivore dieters' | Life and style | The Guardian (no date). Available at: https://www. theguardian.com/lifeandstyle/2018/may/11/the-carnivore-diet-all-meat-health-benefits-dangers (Accessed: 9 March 2019).

11 Nelson, K. M., Dahlin, J. L., Bisson, J., Graham, J., Pauli, G. F. and Walters, M. A. (2017) 'The Essential Medicinal Chemistry of Curcumin', Journal of Medicinal Chemistry, 60(5), pp. 1620 1637. doi: 10.1021/acs.jmedchem.6b00975.

12 Background | Calerie (no date). Available at: https://calerie.duke.edu/ about-the-study/background (Accessed: 9 March 2019).

13 Hallberg, S. J., McKenzie, A. L., Williams, P. T., Bhanpuri, N. H., Peters, A. L., Campbell, W. W., Hazbun, T. L., Volk, B. M., McCarter, J. P., Phinney, S. D. and Volek, J. S. (2018) 'Effectiveness and Safety of a Novel Care Model for the Management of Type 2 Diabetes at 1 Year: An Open-Label, Non-Randomized, Controlled Study', Diabetes Therapy. Springer Healthcare, 9(2), pp. 583–612. doi: 10.1007/ s13300-018-0373-9.

14 Beharry, S. and Heinrich, M. (2018) 'Is the hype around the reproductive health claims of maca (Lepidium meyenii Walp.) justified?', Journal of Ethnopharmacology, 211, pp. 126–170. doi: 10.1016/j.jep.2017.08.003.

15 Houston, M. C., Cooil, B., Olafsson, B. J. and Raggi, P. (2007) 'Juice Powder Concentrate and Systemic Blood Pressure, Progression of Coronary Artery Calcium and Antioxidant Status in Hypertensive Subjects: A Pilot Study', Evidence-Based Complementary and Alternative Medicine, 4(4), pp. 455–462. doi: 10.1093/ecam/nel108.

16 Inserra, P. F., Jiang, S., Solkoff, D., Lee, J., Zhang, Z., Xu, M., Hesslink, R., Wise, J. and Watson, R. R. (1999) 'Immune Function in Elderly Smokers and Nonsmokers Improves During Supplementation with Fruit and Vegetable Extracts', Integrative Medicine. Elsevier, 2(1), pp. 3–10. doi: 10.1016/S1096-2190(99)00010-4.

17 Juice Plus | Cancer Network (no date). Available at: https://www. cancernetwork.com/integrative-oncology/juice-plus (Accessed: 9 March 2019).

18 Juice Plus+® Omega Blend (no date). Available at: https://www. juiceplus.com/gb/en/shop/capsules/omega-blends (Accessed: 9 March 2019).

19 Joseph, R., Giovinazzo, M. and Brown, M. (2016) 'A Literature Review

on the Practice of Placentophagia', Nursing for Women's Health, 20(5), pp. 476–483. doi:10.1016/j.nwh.2016.08.005.

20 Young, S. M., Gryder, L. K., David, W. B., Teng, Y., Gerstenberger, S. and Benyshek, D. C. (2016) 'Human placenta processed for encapsulation contains modest concentrations of 14 trace minerals and elements', Nutrition Research, 36(8), pp. 872–878. doi:10.1016/j.nutres.2016.04.005.

21 Gryder, L. K., Young, S. M., Zava, D., Norris, W., Cross, C. L. and Benyshek, D. C. (2017) 'Effects of Human Maternal Placentophagy on Maternal Postpartum Iron Status: A Randomized, Double-Blind, Placebo-Controlled Pilot Study', Journal of Midwifery & Women's Health, 62(1), pp. 68–79. doi: 10.1111/jmwh.12549.

22 Shaikh, F. H. and Bilquees, S. (2018) 'Placentophagia: Revolution in Postpartum Medicine, or Just a Trend?', Journal of Obstetrics and Gynaecology Canada, 40(3), p. 286. doi: 10.1016/j.jogc.2017.10.009.

Chapter 14 Exploring Evidence

1 Schell, L. M., Gallo, M. V and Cook, K. (2012) 'What's NOT to eat--food adulteration in the context of human biology.', American journal of human biology : the official journal of the Human Biology Council. NIH Public Access, 24(2), pp. 139–48. doi:10.1002/ajhb.22202.

Index